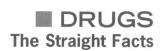

■ DRUGS
The Straight Facts

Diet Pills

DRUGS The Straight Facts

Alcohol

Antidepressants

Body Enhancement Products

Cocaine

Date Rape Drugs

Designer Drugs

Diet Pills

Ecstasy

Hallucinogens

Heroin

Inhalants

Marijuana

Nicotine

Prescription Pain Relievers

Ritalin and Other Methylphenidate-Containing Drugs

Sleep Aids

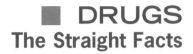

■ DRUGS
The Straight Facts

Diet Pills

Debra Henn
and
Deborah DeEugenio

Consulting Editor
David J. Triggle
University Professor
School of Pharmacy and Pharmaceutical Sciences
State University of New York at Buffalo

"PJC PENSACOLA CAMPUS LRC

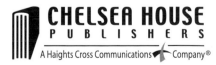

CHELSEA HOUSE
P U B L I S H E R S
A Haights Cross Communications ✦ Company®
P h i l a d e l p h i a

CHELSEA HOUSE PUBLISHERS
VP, New Product Development Sally Cheney
Director of Production Kim Shinners
Creative Manager Takeshi Takahashi
Manufacturing Manager Diann Grasse

Staff for DIET PILLS
Executive Editor Tara Koellhoffer
Associate Editor Beth Reger
Editorial Assistant Kuorkor Dzani
Production Editor Noelle Nardone
Photo Editor Sarah Bloom
Series & Cover Designer Terry Mallon
Layout 21st Century Publishing and Communications, Inc.

A Haights Cross Communications ↞ Company®

http://www.chelseahouse.com

First Printing

1 3 5 7 9 8 6 4 2

Library of Congress Cataloging-in-Publication Data

Henn, Debra.
    Diet pills / Debra Henn and Deborah DeEugenio.
      p. cm.—(Drugs, the straight facts)
Includes bibliographical references.
    ISBN 0-7910-8198-2—ISBN 0-7910-8342-X (pbk.)
  1. Appetite depressants—Popular works. I. DeEugenio, Deborah. II. Title.
III. Series.
RM332.3.H46 2005
615'.78—dc22
                                                    2004024766

All links and web addresses were checked and verified to be correct at the time
of publication. Because of the dynamic nature of the web, some addresses and
links may have changed since publication and may no longer be valid.

Table of Contents

The Use and Abuse of Drugs

The issues associated with drug use and abuse in contemporary society are vexing subjects, fraught with political agendas and ideals that often obscure essential information that teens need to know to have intelligent discussions about how to best deal with the problems associated with drug use and abuse. *Drugs: The Straight Facts* aims to provide this essential information through straightforward explanations of how an individual drug or group of drugs works in both therapeutic and non-therapeutic conditions; with historical information about the use and abuse of specific drugs; with discussion of drug policies in the United States; and with an ample list of further reading.

From the start, the series uses the word *"drug"* to describe psychoactive substances that are used for medicinal or non-medicinal purposes. Included in this broad category are substances that are legal or illegal. It is worth noting that humans have used many of these substances for hundreds, if not thousands of years. For example, traces of marijuana and cocaine have been found in Egyptian mummies; the use of peyote and Amanita fungi has long been a component of religious ceremonies worldwide; and alcohol production and consumption have been an integral part of many human cultures' social and religious ceremonies. One can speculate about why early human societies chose to use such drugs. Perhaps, anything that could provide relief from the harshness of life—anything that could make the poor conditions and fatigue associated with hard work easier to bear—was considered a welcome tonic. Life was likely to be, according to the seventeenth century English philosopher Thomas Hobbes, *"poor, nasty, brutish and short."* One can also speculate about modern human societies' continued use and abuse of drugs. Whatever the reasons, the consequences of sustained drug use are not insignificant—addiction, overdose, incarceration, and drug wars—and must be dealt with by an informed citizenry.

The problem that faces our society today is how to break

the connection between our demand for drugs and the willingness of largely outside countries to supply this highly profitable trade. This is the same problem we have faced since narcotics and cocaine were outlawed by the Harrison Narcotic Act of 1914, and we have yet to defeat it despite current expenditures of approximately $20 billion per year on "the war on drugs." The first step in meeting any challenge is always an intelligent and informed citizenry. The purpose of this series is to educate our readers so that they can make informed decisions about issues related to drugs and drug abuse.

SUGGESTED ADDITIONAL READING

David T. Courtwright, *Forces of Habit. Drugs and the Making of the Modern World.* Cambridge, Mass.: Harvard University Press, 2001. David Courtwright is Professor of History at the University of North Florida.

Richard Davenport-Hines, *The Pursuit of Oblivion. A Global History of Narcotics.* New York: Norton, 2002. The author is a professional historian and a member of the Royal Historical Society.

Aldous Huxley, *Brave New World.* New York: Harper & Row, 1932. Huxley's book, written in 1932, paints a picture of a cloned society devoted only to the pursuit of happiness.

David J. Triggle, Ph.D.
University Professor
School of Pharmacy and Pharmaceutical Sciences
State University of New York at Buffalo

1

The Obesity Epidemic

Hello. My name is Gina, I'm 17 years old, and I weigh 340 pounds (155 kg). I've been overweight since I was 12 years old. I used to go to school, but I dropped out because people make fun of me. I have missed my entire time in high school because of being obese.

I suffer from depression, anxiety, and a fear of leaving my house. I hate my body so much it's insane. I wish I could lose all this weight in a heartbeat, but I know it is not possible. All I am able to do is sit around in the house all day. When I do go out, I can't bring myself to get out of the car. I joined a gym, but I don't know what good that's going to do; I am too embarrassed even to go.

I feel so guilty for letting myself get so big. I wish I could just live an ordinary teenage life and have cute boys look at me and not pick on me. I wish I could go out and enjoy life instead of being afraid all the time. I wish I could simply go to a store and buy sexy clothing, bell-bottoms, tank tops, and a bikini, but I can't because they don't make that kind of clothing in my size.

I know I'm not the only obese person in the world, but being a teenager and watching all these other skinny teenage girls makes me feel like I am the only [obese] one. I feel like such a freak. I wish I could change, but it's so hard. I really need some support right now. I wish all these pretty, skinny, in-shape people could just respect me, but that will never happen because of the way I look.

(Story adapted from an excerpt on the American Obesity Association Website, *http://www.obesity.org/subs/story*)

This is one of the many stories that describe how an adolescent feels when he or she is obese. Overweight and obesity are growing problems. These conditions have reached epidemic proportions in the United States and in most industrialized nations around the world. An explosion in the variety and availability of high-calorie, high-fat convenience foods and the fact that people are exercising less and performing less manual labor have added to the problem. All of the social stigmas involved with being overweight may lead to improper use of aids designed to decrease weight. Once they have decided to lose weight, adolescents, just like adults, want to lose excess weight as quickly as possible and may do so in ways that are not healthy and do not lead to maintenance of weight loss over a long period of time.

DEFINITION OF OVERWEIGHT AND OBESITY

Most people believe someone is obese if they look "fat." This is not true. Health-care professionals and scientists have developed specific definitions for the words *overweight* and *obese*. Overweight and obesity are not determined solely by an individual's weight, but are defined in terms of a person's weight relative to his or her height. Doctors and researchers use a special set of measurements and mathematical formulas to determine whether a person is overweight or obese.

BODY MASS INDEX (BMI)

The body mass index (BMI) is a number calculated from a person's weight and height that can be used to estimate his or her level of body fat. A person is classified as healthy, overweight, or obese based on his or her BMI. The BMI value can be helpful in assessing the health risks a person may face because he or she is carrying too much weight.

A person's BMI is reported as kg/m^2 (Figure 1.1). Adults with a BMI of 25 to 29.9 kg/m^2 are considered overweight. Adults with a BMI over 30 kg/m^2 are considered obese. Being

Are you overweight or obese?

The Body Mass Index (BMI) is used to determine whether a person is at a healthy weight, overweight or obese. BMI has some limitations, in that it can overestimate body fat in people who are very muscular and it can underestimate body fat in people who have lost muscle mass, such as many elderly.

Calculating your BMI   Body Mass Index (BMI) $= \dfrac{\text{Weight (pounds)}}{\text{Height (inches)}^2} \times 703$

Body Mass Index (BMI) chart

Key   ☐ Healthy weight (Below 25)   ☐ Overweight (25-29)   ◼ Obese (30+)

Weight in pounds

Height	120	130	140	150	160	170	180	190	200	210	220	230	240	250
4'6	29	31	34	36	39	41	43	46	48	51	53	56	58	60
4'8	27	29	31	34	36	38	40	43	45	47	49	52	54	56
4'10	25	27	29	31	34	36	38	40	42	44	46	48	50	52
5'0	23	25	27	29	31	33	35	37	39	41	43	45	47	49
5'2	22	24	26	27	29	31	33	35	37	38	40	42	44	46
5'4	21	22	24	26	28	29	31	33	34	36	38	40	41	43
5'6	19	21	23	24	26	27	29	31	32	34	36	37	39	40
5'8	18	20	21	23	24	26	27	29	30	32	34	35	37	38
5'10	17	19	20	22	23	24	26	27	29	30	32	33	35	36
6'0	16	18	19	20	22	23	24	26	27	28	30	31	33	34
6'2	15	17	18	19	21	22	23	24	26	27	28	30	31	32
6'4	15	16	17	18	20	21	22	23	24	26	27	28	29	30
6'6	14	15	16	17	19	20	21	22	23	24	25	27	28	29
6'8	13	14	15	17	18	19	20	21	22	23	24	25	26	28

NOTE: Chart is for adults aged 20 and older.

SOURCE: Office of the Surgeon General   AP

Figure 1.1 The body mass index (BMI) is a formula that calculates whether a person is an ideal body weight, overweight, or obese. The formula used to calculate BMI considers a person's weight and height. BMI has some limitations. It may not be accurate for people who are very muscular, such as bodybuilders, and people with very little muscle mass, such as the elderly. BMI is one of several factors health-care providers consider when they determine whether a person is overweight or obese. Note that this BMI chart is designed for adults who are age 20 or older.

overweight and obese are not mutually exclusive; all obese individuals are also considered overweight.

A measurement called the *percentile of BMI* is used to identify overweight and obesity in children and adolescents. The Centers for Disease Control and Prevention (CDC), an organization that defines the healthy height and weight information for growing children that is found on national growth charts, avoids using the word *obesity* for children and adolescents. The CDC chooses not to use the word *obese* because children are still growing and may "grow into" their weight. Instead, the CDC suggests two levels into which overweight or obese children can be placed:

1. The 85th percentile, defining those who are at risk for becoming obese.

2. The 95th percentile, the more severe level used to describe children who are already obese.

BMI (and percentile of BMI) is only one factor in determining a person's weight-related health risk. Having a BMI in the "healthy" range does not necessarily mean that a person is fit and healthy. BMI does not take into account lean body mass or body frame. A muscular, large-framed person's BMI could indicate that he or she is obese, but other factors would show that this is not the case.

The presence of excess fat in the stomach area is also a negative factor to be considered in overweight individuals. People who have fat in the abdomen that is out of proportion to their total body fat have what is called *central obesity*. A person with central obesity is defined as having a circumference, or distance around the waist, of greater than 40 inches in adult men and greater than 35 inches in adult women. Studies have shown that people with central obesity have a higher risk of weight-related health problems than do people whose body fat is more evenly distributed. The reason for this is not known, but health studies have shown that there is a significant increase in heart problems in people with central obesity.

HEALTH RISKS ASSOCIATED WITH OBESITY

Obesity is currently the second leading cause of preventable death in the United States.[1] Being overweight and obese can contribute to death by causing or worsening many different diseases, including but not limited to:

- High blood pressure;

- High cholesterol (overweight individuals often have higher levels of "bad" cholesterol and lower levels of "good" cholesterol);

- Obstructive sleep apnea (a condition where a person may stop breathing for a period of time while sleeping);

- Rheumatoid arthritis and osteoarthritis;

- Certain types of cancer, including breast, esophageal, stomach, colorectal, endometrial, and kidney cancer;

- In women: menstrual disturbances, infertility problems, and an increased incidence of birth defects in children;

- Increased daytime sleepiness and heat intolerance;

- Obesity may also contribute to gallbladder disease, gout, breathing problems, increased incidence of infections, liver diseases, and increased pain, especially in the lower back and knees.

Two of the biggest health problems that overweight individuals face are a greatly elevated risk of heart disease and stroke. The American Heart Association (AHA) has found a direct link between these health conditions and being overweight. Heart disease is now the number-one killer of women in the United States, and the rise of overweight and obesity can be directly correlated to it.[2]

A person's risk of developing these health conditions increases as his or her BMI increases, so obese individuals are at higher risk than overweight individuals. Weight loss of even 10 to 15 pounds (4.5 to 6.8 kg) in adults and children can decrease the risk of developing health problems such as diabetes and hypertension. This weight loss can also help to control or lessen the severity of these conditions in patients already afflicted with these conditions. As previously noted, adults with central obesity are at higher risk of developing many of these conditions than are people with evenly distributed body fat.

Obese children also have an increased incidence of health problems. As the prevalence of obesity has increased in children, there has been a similar rise in diseases that were previously rare in children, including type II diabetes and hypertension (high blood pressure). There is a high incidence of obesity among children with asthma, which may indicate a link between the two conditions. There is also an increase in bone and joint complications in obese children. During childhood, bone and cartilage is still growing and developing, and is not strong enough to bear excess weight.

OBESITY THROUGH THE AGES

As far back as ancient Egypt, being overweight was a sign of wealth, not a sign that a person lacked self-control. People in the early 16th century dined on avocados, chili peppers, milk, and potatoes—a diet very high in fat. As recently as the 1950s, famous stars like Marilyn Monroe were not considered overweight, but wore a size 12 and had the kind of curves every woman wanted. Fast-forward to the Hollywood stars of today—like Halle Berry and Heather Locklear—and you see thin and seemingly "perfect" women who reflect a wholesale change in how beauty is perceived and defined in our culture.

SOCIAL ISSUES ASSOCIATED WITH OBESITY

Anyone who has watched an episode of *Friends* or *The OC* has seen the glorified ideal of being thin; the characters are extremely thin and ultimately many people who watch the show are inclined to want to lose weight, even if they do so in harmful ways. Unrealistic and unhealthy ideals of thinness are presented everywhere in the media—particularly in movies, television, and magazines. These images compel many people to try tactics (both conventional and unconventional) to lose weight, firm up, and match these ideals.

In large part because of the "thinner is better" message put forth by the media, obese individuals experience social and emotional stress because of their weight. In the United States, Canada, and other Westernized societies, there are powerful messages that people should be thin and that overweight individuals have poor self-control. Negative attitudes toward obese people may lead to discrimination in employment or college acceptance, even though this kind of discrimination is illegal. Some obese people, particularly adolescents, may experience an increased incidence of depression and emotional stress. Teens may also have a poor self-image and feelings of isolation, as well as directed messages of negativity from peers.

OBESITY TRENDS IN THE UNITED STATES

It is estimated that 50% of adults in the United States are overweight, with approximately half of those falling into the obese category. The prevalence of obesity in adults has increased approximately 60% in the United States between the years 1991 and 2001. (Figure 1.2)[3]

Studies show that children are getting heavier as time goes on. A comparison of childhood obesity studies completed in 1961 against similar studies completed today revealed that the incidence of childhood obesity has doubled. This trend exposes an ever-increasing number of children both to the societal impacts of being overweight and to a number of

More obesity in land of plenty

The percentage of Americans who are obese has risen since 1991. The increase cuts across all ages, racial and ethnic groups and both genders. About 300,000 deaths each year are associated with obesity.

Percent of obese U.S. adults

☐ No data   ☐ Less than 10%   ☐ 10-14%   ☐ 15-19%   ■ 20%+

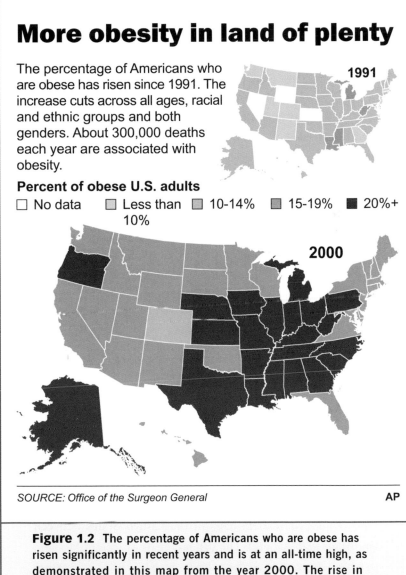

SOURCE: Office of the Surgeon General   AP

Figure 1.2 The percentage of Americans who are obese has risen significantly in recent years and is at an all-time high, as demonstrated in this map from the year 2000. The rise in obesity is seen in males and females of all ages, including children. This increase in obesity has also been seen in all racial and ethnic groups. The increase in obesity is attributed to decreased exercise and manual labor, along with consumption of larger portions of high-calorie, high-fat foods.

potentially serious health problems, not the least of which are diabetes, high blood pressure, and asthma.

In the United States, approximately 30% of children and adolescents ages 6 to 19 are overweight and 15% are obese. Children and adolescents who are overweight are more likely to be overweight as adults. Overweight children ages 10 to 14 who have at least one overweight or obese parent were reported to have an almost 80% chance of remaining over-weight as they enter adulthood.[4]

Obesity tends to be most prevalent among certain groups, such as specific minority groups, people with low incomes, and people with less education. In some cases, people within a certain ethnic group may be taught traditional methods of cooking that are high in fat (for example, frying chicken instead of baking it). Certain cultures more readily accept larger body types and therefore do not have a negative view of obesity. People with less education are less likely to know the health risks associated with obesity, and therefore have a higher rate of this condition.

With the high prevalence and steady increase in over-weight and obesity in the United States comes a steady increase in the use of various diet supplements, including both non-prescription and prescription diet pills.

PREVENTION AND TREATMENT OF OBESITY: WEIGHT LOSS GOALS

There is strong evidence that weight loss in overweight and obese individuals decreases their risk of diseases, such as heart conditions and diabetes. The general goals of weight loss and management are to reduce body weight, prevent further weight gain, and maintain a lower body weight over the long term. The initial goal of weight loss in an obese person should be to lose 10% of total body weight, which is manageable for most obese individuals. Once achieved, the 10% weight loss is often easy to maintain. For example, a 300-pound (136-kg) person should initially strive to lose 30 pounds (66 kg). This weight loss should occur over approximately six months. The target should be lose ž to 2 lbs (0.2 to 1 kg) per week to achieve the initial weight loss goal over six months. Studies have proven that this seemingly small amount of weight loss can have a substantial effect on lowering the risk of developing or worsening diabetes and heart disease. After six months, tactics to maintain weight loss should be put into place. If more weight loss is needed, another attempt at weight reduction can be made. Adults should work to attain a BMI lower than 25 kg/m². Any additional decrease in BMI, however, will reduce the overall health risks. It is best for individuals to consult their doctor or health-care professional before embarking on any weight loss plan.

STRATEGIES FOR WEIGHT LOSS AND WEIGHT MAINTENANCE

This chapter has focused mainly on the statistics and health risks related to obesity and overweight. General approaches to weight loss include changing the diet and getting more exercise. Watching portion size is one of the first strategies a person can adopt to help reach a weight-loss goal. Also available for people looking to lose weight is a wide variety of reduced-fat and low-calorie foods. Like other foods, these products must be eaten in moderation, but they offer an option that can easily be substituted into a person's everyday diet. Finally, simple behavioral changes can help a person lose weight. Walking up a flight of stairs instead of using the elevator is exercise that can easily be incorporated into a person's daily routine. There are many other ways that weight loss can occur; some of these strategies will be discussed in greater detail in later chapters.

WHEN ARE DIET PILLS RECOMMENDED?

The question of when and how diet pills should be used will be examined in later chapters. Overall, in carefully selected patients, a doctor may prescribe appropriate drugs to be used in conjunction with diet and exercise to achieve weight loss. The only drugs recommended for use by the National Heart, Lung, and Blood Institute (NHLBI) are those that have been approved by the U.S. Food and Drug Administration (FDA). FDA-approved drugs have been studied and determined to be safe and effective for some, but not all, people. These drugs and the selection process will be discussed in more detail in Chapter 4.

According to the NHLBI, people who are appropriate candidates and should consider taking diet pills are adults with a BMI of greater than 30 kg/m^2 or those with a BMI of higher than 27 kg/m^2 who have health problems related to being overweight. Diet pills, like any other medication, have risks associated with their use. Therefore, diet pills should only be used by people who are at high risk of developing weight-related health problems. For people who are obese or overweight, the benefits of weight loss are generally greater than the risks associated with taking diet pills. Several diet pills have been studied for use in children; however, doctors only recommend using them in extreme situations.

The National Institutes of Health (NIH) has established guidelines on the use of diet pills. These guidelines are used by health-care practitioners both within and outside the United States. The information contained in these guidelines helps to determine who should and should not use weight loss medications. This is important because people who use diet pills inappropriately risk potentially devastating effects on their health.

2

Causes of Obesity

In general mankind, since the improvement of cookery, eats twice as much as nature requires.

—Benjamin Franklin,
American scientist, publisher, and diplomat

There is a simple equation that explains how a person's body maintains its weight. To maintain a steady body weight, the amount of energy a person takes in (the number of calories he or she eats) must equal the amount of energy the person uses (how many calories he or she burns). To lose weight, a person must shift the balance of the energy equation so that the amount of energy coming in is less than the amount of energy going out (Figure 2.1). This can be achieved by reducing the amount of energy taken in (that is, eating fewer calories), increasing the amount of energy used (for example, by exercising), or by combining the two strategies (diet and exercise). Unfortunately, for millions of Americans, the energy taken in is far greater than the energy used. This extra energy is stored in their bodies as fat, resulting in weight gain.

The human body is designed to take in and process the amount of energy it needs to perform daily activities. If the body takes in more calories than it needs, it stores these calories as adipose tissue, or fat, for later use. In earlier times, this storage of calories by the body helped people survive through periods when little or no food was available (famine). During times of famine, the body burned its fat stores to obtain the energy it needed to perform normal activities. If people did not have these fat stores, they would starve during times when less food was available.

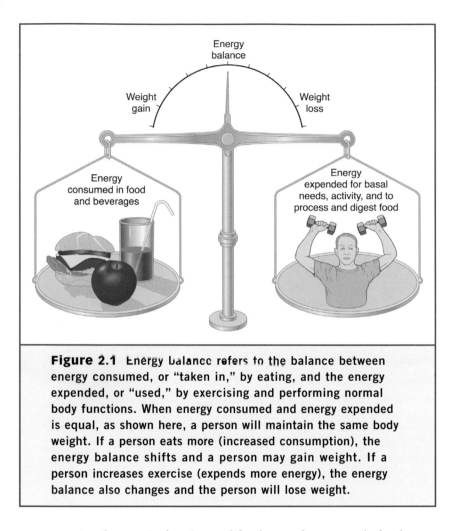

Figure 2.1 Energy balance refers to the balance between energy consumed, or "taken in," by eating, and the energy expended, or "used," by exercising and performing normal body functions. When energy consumed and energy expended is equal, as shown here, a person will maintain the same body weight. If a person eats more (increased consumption), the energy balance shifts and a person may gain weight. If a person increases exercise (expends more energy), the energy balance also changes and the person will lose weight.

As advances in farming and food manufacture made food more plentiful in many parts of the world, the need for fat stores in the body decreased. People continued to eat more calories than they needed, though, and their bodies continued to store it as fat (Figure 2.2) that was not needed and would not likely be used. It is this accumulation of fat stores that has led to the problem of obesity. Whereas in the past people would likely burn off their fat stores during times of famine, in today's world they need to make a conscious effort

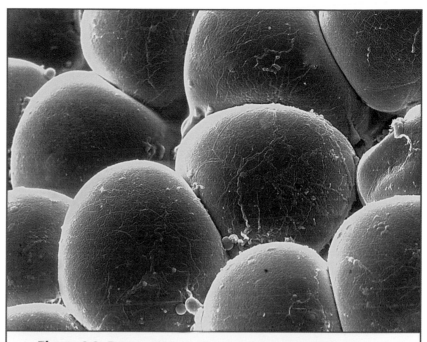

Figure 2.2 Fat, or adipose, cells store extra energy from food. Adipose cells help insulate the body to keep it warm, cushion and protect the internal organs, and store extra energy for later use. When people consume more energy from food, the extra energy is stored as fat in adipose cells. Years ago, this stored energy could be used to avoid starvation in times of famine. Today, people never use this stored fat because famine does not exist in developed countries. These fat cells continue to accumulate and lead to weight gain and eventually to obesity.

to increase physical activity or decrease the calories they consume if they want to lose weight.

FACTORS THAT CONTRIBUTE TO OBESITY

Why are some people obese and some are not? It is not acceptable in most Western cultures to be obese; therefore, most people attempt to maintain an average weight (as discussed in Chapter 1). What predisposes certain people to become obese?

Overweight and obesity are caused by a combination of genetic and environmental factors. Some people have a genetic predisposition to gain weight and store fat. For others, the factors that lead to obesity can be found in the world they inhabit and the behaviors they choose.

Genetics

Genetics clearly play a role in obesity. It has been noted that an adopted child's body weight is usually more similar to the body weight of his or her biological parents than that of his or her adopted parents. Identical twins usually have similar occurrences of obesity. Studies have also shown that fraternal twins do not show this same likelihood of obesity; when one twin is overweight, the other is very often not. These examples help demonstrate that genetics play a significant role in obesity.

Researchers participating in the Human Obesity Gene Map project are in the early stages of determining which genes contribute to obesity in people. Several alterations in normal genes have been discovered in laboratory rodents and linked to obesity in these animals. These genes include the *ob* or *lep* gene and the *Agouti* gene. Researchers are working to find out if these same genes contribute to obesity in humans.

Not all people who have obesity genes will be overweight. Conversely, some people who are overweight will not have these genes. This is because environmental factors also play a major role in causing overweight and obesity.

Environmental Factors

Along with genetics, environmental factors have been found to contribute to obesity. In particular, increased food consumption and an inactive (sedentary) lifestyle are environmental factors that very closely correlate with an increased risk of obesity.

Americans have an ever-increasing number of energy-dense foods, packaged in enormous portions, conveniently available at low cost. Energy-dense foods contain large numbers of calories in very small portions. These foods promote the overconsumption of calories. Americans also consume 40% of their calories from fats, which is well above the level recommended by the American Heart Association (AHA). Fats are an extremely energy-dense form of nutrition. The AHA recommends that adults obtain less than 30% of their daily calories from fat.

In the United States and in other developed countries, modern technology allows people to be less active in their daily tasks, since many things today are automated and do not require manual labor. For example, years ago people walked to most places. Today, people have access to cars and public transportation to take them to these same places, thus limiting the need for physical activity.

Decreases in physical activity can lead to weight gain. Ultimately, all the calories you eat are not utilized, or burned off. Calories that are not utilized are stored as fat tissue, which

OBESITY GENES

The *ob* or *lep* gene codes for a protein called leptin. Rats with an alteration in this gene have less leptin produced in their bodies. These rats eat more than rats that have normal amounts of leptin. Leptin may cause an increase in insulin, a hormone in the body that is associated with weight gain when present in high amounts. When the rats with the altered *ob* or *lep* genes were injected with leptin, they ate less and produced normal amounts of insulin, suggesting that the missing leptin may be the cause of their obesity. Researchers believe that obese humans may also have an alteration in this gene, and they are now working to develop a form of leptin that could be put into a diet pill for human use. It will take many years to determine if such a pill would be safe and effective.

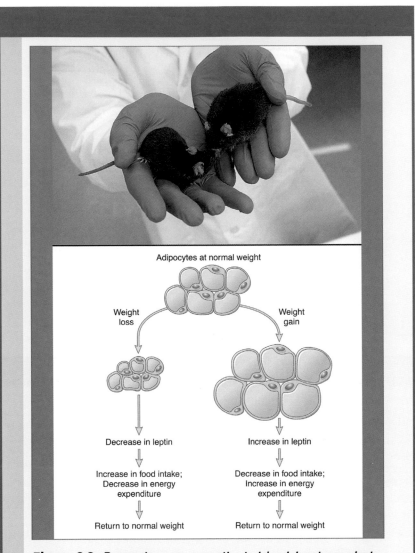

Figure 2.3 *Researchers are currently studying laboratory rodents, like the mice in the upper photograph, to try to identify specific genes that may lead to obesity. The two mice shown are the same, except that the mouse on the left has had one gene removed. As you can see, the mouse on the left is thin, while the mouse on the right is obese. This leads researchers to believe that the gene removed may help cause obesity. By better understanding the causes of obesity, researchers will be better able to develop treatments for this condition in humans.*

can lead to weight gain. Sedentary behavior is on the rise now that technology and automation are so widely available. All of the modern conveniences we now have accessible to us have eliminated the need for individuals to perform much of the physical activity that was once required for daily tasks at work and home (Table 2.1). Computers, cable and satellite television, movies on demand, and high-tech toys like video game systems have led to a decrease in physical activity in people of all ages. Reduced physical education requirements in schools across the nation have also caused physical activity to decline among adolescents. The CDC estimates that 70% of adults in the United States fail to meet minimal recommendations for physical activity. It also estimates that about one-third of people over the age of 18 get no leisure-time physical activity at all.

Other environmental factors that have been linked to obesity are lower economic class, lower education level, and cessation (quitting) of smoking. The link between economic level, educational background, and obesity is not clear. One theory is that a person who is illiterate may not be able to read labels on food and may not be aware he or she is consuming high-fat, high-calorie foods that can lead to obesity. High-fat, high-calorie foods, such as the food served at most fast-food restaurants, are formulated to be cheap and great tasting. This food is readily available and affordable for people with lower incomes and it is speculated that these people may consume more of this type of food, which can lead to obesity (Figure 2.4).

People who quit smoking are also likely to gain weight and potentially become obese. It is believed that the nicotine withdrawal a person experiences when he or she quits smoking causes an increase in appetite that leads to an increased intake of calories and, thus, weight gain. This trade-off is not an easy one to handle. The harmful effects of smoking are many and include lung cancer, bronchitis (an infection of the tube that brings air to the lungs), and emphysema (a condition that

THE NUMBER OF CALORIES IN FAST FOODS

The average person should consume 15 calories per pound of body weight each day. For example, a 130-pound person should consume 1,950 calories each day (15 calories/pound x 130 lbs = 1,950 calories). Approximately 30% of those calories should come from fat (1,950 calories x 0.30 = 585 calories/day). To illustrate the huge number of calories contained in the energy-dense fast food that is conveniently available, let's consider a standard meal from a popular fast-food chain[a]:

	TOTAL CALORIES	FAT CALORIES
Double Cheeseburger	600	300
Large French Fries	520	230
Large Cola	310	0
Total	1,430	530

The 130-pound person in our example should consume 1,950 total daily calories, with 585 calories coming from fat. You can see that this one meal contains 75% of the calories and 90% of the fat calories this person needs for the entire day. If this person eats three meals a day like this one, he or she will consume close to three times the calories his or her body requires. The vast majority of these calories will wind up being stored as fat.

Source: a. Nutrition Facts for McDonald's restaurants. Available online at http://www.mcdonalds.com.

results in labored breathing and increased risk of infections). Many people who quit smoking trade one health risk (smoking) for another (obesity) because they gain weight. Rimonabant, a drug that is currently being studied, may be able to help a person quit smoking and lose weight at the same time. Until this drug is released, however, smoking cessation

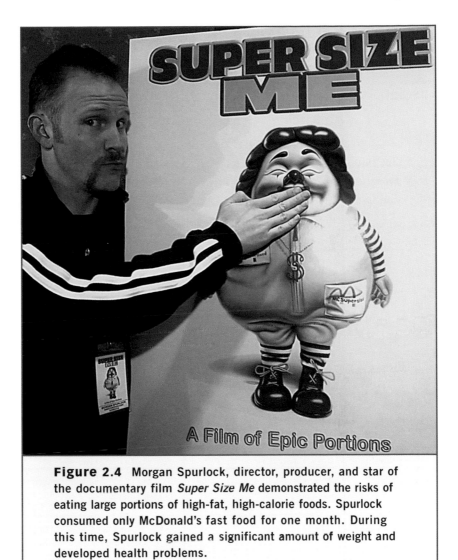

Figure 2.4 Morgan Spurlock, director, producer, and star of the documentary film *Super Size Me* demonstrated the risks of eating large portions of high-fat, high-calorie foods. Spurlock consumed only McDonald's fast food for one month. During this time, Spurlock gained a significant amount of weight and developed health problems.

and the weight gain that can come with it must be handled with dietary changes and exercise.

Drugs and Hormones

Several drugs and hormones have an effect on body weight. Some hormones cause weight gain and others cause weight

Table 2.1 How Modernization Has Impacted Obesity by Decreasing Physical Activity

Transportation:	More people own cars	Fewer people are walking and riding bicycles, even for short distances
In the Home:	Modern appliances, such as microwaves, dishwashers, washing machines, and vacuum cleaners, are more prevalent	People perform less manual labor at home, such as washing clothes and dishes, and cleaning floors by hand
	Pre-packaged foods and frozen or "quick-prepare" dinners are increasingly available and appealing to time-stressed consumers	Increase in consumption of "convenience foods" that are often high in fat and calories and low in nutritional value
	Individuals spend more time watching television, playing video games, and using the computer	Decrease in active sports and exercise
At Work:	Technolgy, such as computers and automated farm and factory equipment, lead to more "desk jobs"	Fewer jobs require manual labor
Public Places:	Use of elevators, escalators, and automated doors	Decrease in physical activity such as stair-climbing
In the Community:	Increase in crime	People are less likely to go outside for leisure and exercise; children are more likely to remain inside after school

loss. Hormones that cause weight gain are of particular interest, because if researchers can study and understand how they work, they may be able to develop drugs that can interact with these hormones in a way that makes it easier for people to lose weight.

Insulin is a hormone that helps turn glucose (the sugar found in food) into energy the body can use. High levels of insulin lead to weight gain, although the reason why is not fully understood. Drugs used to treat diabetes, such as insulin and medications that make the body produce more insulin, cause weight gain. Obese people often have higher levels of naturally occurring insulin than their leaner counterparts.

Female hormones, like progesterone and estrogen, are associated with weight gain. Obese women most commonly begin to gain weight after puberty, when their bodies begin to produce these hormones. Birth control pills contain estrogen and progesterone, and are associated with weight gain. Today, birth control pills cause less weight gain than in previous years because they contain lower levels of estrogen. Some women may gain more weight than usual during pregnancy, up to 110 pounds (50 kg), which may be related to differences in their hormone levels during pregnancy, as compared to other pregnant women. Women who gain excessive weight during pregnancy may never fully lose this weight. Changes in hormone levels also occur during menopause. These hormone changes lead to a change in fat distribution, including increased central obesity (fat around the midsection or waist). This fat distribution is associated with increased health risks, especially heart disease.

Thyroid hormones increase metabolism and cause weight loss. People with the disease hypothyroidism (under-activity of the thyroid gland) have a smaller amount of thyroid hormone. People with hypothyroidism are predisposed to weight gain. When these individuals are treated with a drug that contains thyroid hormones, they lose weight. Thyroid hormones are dangerous in very high levels and must be monitored closely when taken. An excess of thyroid hormones in the blood can lead to several health problems, including high blood pressure, nervousness, insomnia (trouble sleeping), menstrual cycle changes, heart palpitations (the feeling that the heart is pounding), and fever.

Several hormones that may play a role in weight gain have recently been discovered. One of these is leptin, a newly discovered hormone produced in fatty tissue. Increased leptin decreases food intake and increases metabolism in rats and, according to some early studies, in humans as well. Other hormones released by the stomach—including neuropeptide Y, cholecystokinin (CCK), enterostatin, and polypeptide Y 3-36—tell the body it has consumed enough food and should stop eating. Another hormone, ghrelin, is produced by the stomach. Ghrelin signals hunger and increases appetite.

JOANNE

Joanne had been feeling tired and noticed a steady weight gain over the past few months. She had gained a total of 20 pounds and was disgusted with herself. Joanne really did not feel she was eating any more than usual, but she continued to gain weight. She was tired all the time and her mother told her she seemed depressed. Joanne's mother took her to the doctor, and the doctor ran some blood tests. Joanne was diagnosed with a condition called hypothyroidism. The doctor explained that Joanne's thyroid gland (located in her neck) was not producing enough thyroid hormone, and that thyroid hormone is needed to maintain proper energy and metabolism. Joanne was prescribed a drug called Synthroid®, which would increase her thyroid hormones to normal levels. The doctor explained that too much thyroid hormone was also harmful, so Joanne had to come back in eight weeks to check her hormone levels again.

Over the next three months, Joanne's energy returned and she lost the 20 pounds she had gained. This is an example of how hormones may affect body weight.

Table 2.2 Hormones that Influence Body Weight

HORMONE	EFFECT
Estrogen	Weight gain
Ghrelin	Weight gain
Insulin	Weight gain
Neuropeptide Y	Weight gain
Progesterone	Weight gain
Cholecystokinin	Weight loss
Leptin	Weight loss
Polypeptide Y 3-36	Weight loss
Thyroid hormones	Weight loss

Ghrelin concentrations increase in response to weight loss. This may make ghrelin partly responsible for people gaining weight back after a successful diet. Table 2.2 lists some of the hormones that influence body weight.

Clearly, many hormones affect body weight. Some of these hormones are known, and some have not yet been discovered. By studying these hormones, researchers can better understand what causes people to gain and lose weight. Eventually, researchers may be able to develop drugs that can change levels of these hormones in the body, thus giving people who are overweight or obese another weapon in the weight loss battle. Intensive study is required to identify the possible negative effects of increasing or decreasing the level of hormones in the body.

3

How Diet Pills Work

In the quest for the perfect diet pill, scientists, doctors, and those who are going to use these drugs need to understand how diet pills work. Knowing what actions a drug takes and how it affects the body helps scientists and doctors understand what side effects the drug may cause. Recognizing side effects and understanding what causes them can, in turn, help researchers formulate drugs with fewer or less serious side effects.

HOW DO DIET PILLS CAUSE WEIGHT LOSS?

Diet pills work by affecting the body processes that cause weight gain. Diet pills work to cause weight loss in one of three main ways:

1. Increasing energy expenditure (calories burned).

2. Decreasing the number of calories that are absorbed during digestion.

3. Suppressing appetite to decrease how much food is eaten.

Increasing Energy Expenditure (Calories Burned)

Calories consumed in food are used by the body as fuel. The body's use of calories as its source of energy is called *thermogenesis*. Literally, *thermogenesis* means "the production of heat" because when people burn calories, heat is produced. The body needs a constant supply of fuel to maintain normal functions that people don't usually think about, like breathing.

Certain drugs cause the body to burn more calories as it performs its normal daily functions. By burning more calories, people lose weight even though they are eating the same amount. These drugs increase the body's fuel requirements, ideally to a point where the body needs more calories than the person takes in from food. When this happens, the body begins breaking down its fat stores as fuel. As these fat stores are used, people lose weight.

Side effects associated with this type of diet pill often occur because, in causing the body to burn more calories, the pills speed up many body processes—possibly to a level that becomes dangerous. Examples are increased blood pressure and heart rate, which can lead to heart problems over time. Other side effects include nervousness and insomnia.

Many diet pills that work by increasing the number of calories burned have been developed. Most of these contain one or more of the three ingredients: caffeine, phenyl-propanolamine (PPA), and ephedrine. In the United States, PPA and ephedrine have been withdrawn from the market because they produce serious side effects, including heart attack and stroke. Caffeine, which is still found in many diet pills, will be further discussed in Chapter 6.

Decreasing Calorie Absorption

After food is eaten, it is digested in the stomach. The digested nutrients from food are absorbed, mainly in the intestines, into the bloodstream and are used as fuel for the body. When people eat more food than they need, the body stores the extra nutrients as fat, which accounts for weight gain.

Some diet drugs are able to prevent the body from absorbing some of the calories contained in food. People who take these drugs can eat the same amount of food and take in the same number of calories and still lose weight, because the drug causes their bodies to absorb and use fewer calories. The excess calories are eliminated in the stool. Drugs that prevent absorption of nutrients in the intestine may also prevent other drugs a person may be taking from being absorbed. For this reason, it is important not to take these diet pills at the same time as other medications, and to separate them by a few hours. Since these drugs affect the digestive system, including the stomach and intestines, they may also lead to side effects like diarrhea and flatulence (passing gas).

Currently, the only drug on the market that works by blocking the body's absorption of calories is orlistat, which is sold under the brand name Xenical®. Orlistat specifically decreases the absorption of fats from food consumed. A further discussion of orlistat and how it works can be found in Chapter 5.

Appetite Suppression

Appetite is controlled by many factors (Figure 3.1). Processes in the body tell people when they are hungry and when they are satiated (full). Neurotransmitters (chemical messengers in the brain) such as norepinephrine, serotonin, and dopamine tell the brain that the stomach feels full (Figure 3.2). Drugs that increase the levels of these neurotransmitters cause a decrease in appetite by relaying the message that the stomach is full, thus telling the brain to send a "stop eating!" signal. These drugs are effective because, in general, appetite decreases when a person feels full. Drugs that increase more than one of the neurotransmitters may be more effective for weight loss than those that increase only one. Some drugs that work in this way also have the effect of increasing the number of calories burned (thermogenesis).

Dopamine, norepinephrine, and serotonin have other responsibilities in the body besides dictating hunger. For example, norepinephrine also helps control blood pressure. Drugs that affect the level of these neurotransmitters interfere with other body processes and produce negative side effects. A drug that increases norepinephrine will decrease appetite, but

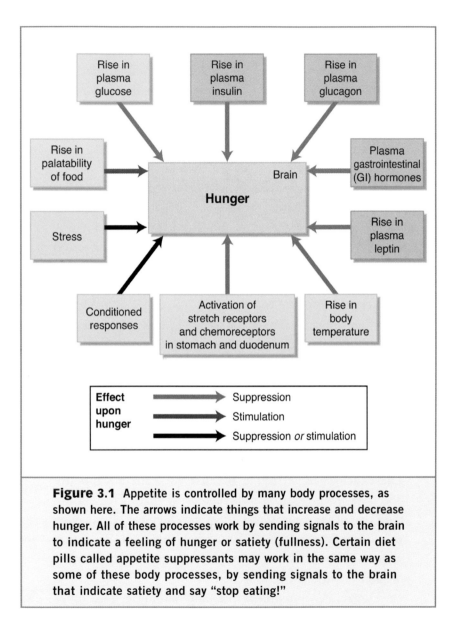

Figure 3.1 Appetite is controlled by many body processes, as shown here. The arrows indicate things that increase and decrease hunger. All of these processes work by sending signals to the brain to indicate a feeling of hunger or satiety (fullness). Certain diet pills called appetite suppressants may work in the same way as some of these body processes, by sending signals to the brain that indicate satiety and say "stop eating!"

will also increase blood pressure. Other common side effects of drugs that increase norepinephrine are dry mouth, insomnia, and constipation. Examples of diet pills that affect these neurotransmitters are sibutramine (Meridia®) and phentermine

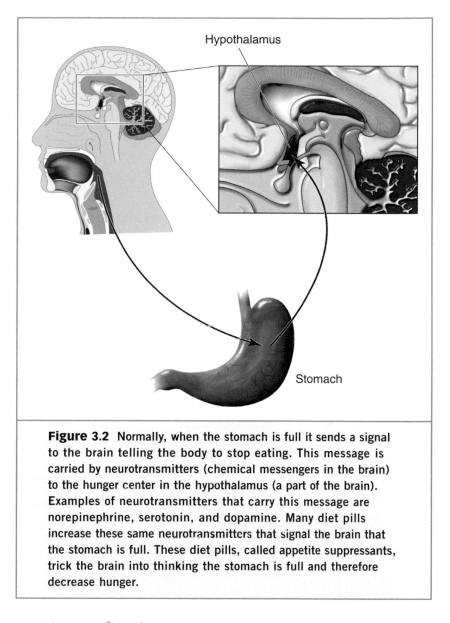

Figure 3.2 Normally, when the stomach is full it sends a signal to the brain telling the body to stop eating. This message is carried by neurotransmitters (chemical messengers in the brain) to the hunger center in the hypothalamus (a part of the brain). Examples of neurotransmitters that carry this message are norepinephrine, serotonin, and dopamine. Many diet pills increase these same neurotransmitters that signal the brain that the stomach is full. These diet pills, called appetite suppressants, trick the brain into thinking the stomach is full and therefore decrease hunger.

(Ionamin®). Sibutramine increases norepinephrine and serotonin. Phentermine increases norepinephrine only.

Other hormones and proteins in the body may also affect appetite. Many of these have been discovered recently and may be useful in the development of new diet pills. As previously discussed, the most promising protein so far is leptin, which is produced by fat stores and tells the body it is full. Several other known proteins and hormones (see Table 2.2 on page 31) affect appetite and may in the future be formulated into drugs for weight loss.

Understanding how hormones work in the body and how they affect satiety (the feeling of being full) is crucial to the development of new products for weight loss. Scientists continue to learn of different processes in the body, even at the cellular level, that can lead to weight gain. Amid the explosion of obesity, scientists continue to identify chemicals with the potential to be turned into drugs that can be used to assist with weight loss, although diet and exercise will always be the best, first-line strategies for losing weight.

4

Diet Pills: The Past

The use of diet aids began around 1900. Since then, many drugs have been used to assist with weight loss. Some of these drugs, while very effective, produced serious side effects. These side effects were often not recognized until many people became sick, or even died.

The U.S. government has taken certain steps in an attempt to ensure the safety and effectiveness of drugs sold in the United States. The U.S. Food and Drug Administration (FDA) began screening drugs for safety in 1938 and effectiveness in 1962. The FDA requires that manufacturers perform studies to prove that their drugs are safe and effective before they may be sold legally in the United States. In 1951, the U.S. government began requiring people to obtain a doctor's prescription before they could take certain medications. This ensured that a physician or other health-care provider was able to examine the patient and determine that the benefits of the drug outweighed any risk of side effects for that individual.

Prior to these government efforts, unsafe drugs were available to the American public. The FDA's laws have greatly improved the safety of available drugs. However, some drugs approved by the FDA are used inappropriately by the public. Drugs that have been judged as safe can become unsafe when used in the wrong way— for example, by being used at too high a dose, for too long a period of time, or in combination with another drug that causes a dangerous interaction. A major problem with diet pills is that people tend to take them for longer than is recommended by the FDA. This is due in part to the fact that people often regain weight when they stop taking diet pills.

The term *dietary supplement* has a specific meaning in the United States that was established by the Dietary Supplement Health and Education Act of 1994 (DSHEA). It refers to a substance that supplements the diet and whose label clearly states that it is a dietary supplement. It is different from a *drug*, which is defined as a substance that is intended to "diagnose, cure, mitigate, treat, or prevent diseases" and which must undergo extensive testing and be approved by the FDA before being sold. Dietary supplements generally contain vitamins, minerals, herbs, other plant-derived substances, amino acids (the individual building blocks of protein), and extracts of these substances.

Natural and herbal diet pills available in the United States today are considered dietary supplements and are not subject to FDA review prior to being sold. Although these agents may have drug-like activity in the body, they do not need to be proven safe or effective like conventional drugs do. Unlike conventional drugs, natural and herbal diet pills can only be withdrawn from the market when they are proven to be dangerous. As a result, many herbal products reach the market without any scientific evidence that they are safe or effective. These products are discussed in more detail in Chapter 6.

As you will see in this chapter, many diet pills that have been available in the United States have produced devastating side effects. The drugs and herbal products discussed in this chapter have been determined to be unsafe and are no longer legally available in the United States for the purpose of weight loss. It is only possible to obtain these drugs by prescription for uses other than weight loss. This is not to say that these drugs cannot still be obtained by a person who is willing to ignore the risks. One way a person might obtain these drugs is on the "black market" (illegally), usually over the Internet.

THYROID HORMONE PILLS
Thyroid hormones are produced in the body by the thyroid

gland. They are necessary for growth, and they stimulate carbohydrate use in the body. It is well known that individuals with an overactive thyroid gland (hyperthyroidism) experience increases in metabolism and carbohydrate use. People with too much thyroid hormone tend to lose 15% of their body weight. This weight is regained when their thyroid is treated and thyroid hormone levels return to normal.

In 1893, thyroid extract was marketed under various brand names, including Frank J. Kellogg's Safe Fat Reducer, Corpulin, and Marmola. People took thyroid hormone pills (or liquid) in addition to having natural thyroid hormones produced by their thyroid glands. The result was an excess of thyroid hormone in the body, which caused increases in metabolism, increased burning of calories, and weight loss.

At the time, the FDA did not evaluate drugs for safety or efficacy prior to their reaching the market. Prescriptions were not required to obtain medications, so people could obtain thyroid hormones at any corner pharmacy or apothecary without being seen by a doctor. Although these thyroid hormone extracts did produce weight loss, they were not safe.

In individuals who took thyroid hormones, 80% of the weight lost was lean body mass (muscle and bone) rather than excess fat. People taking these extracts experienced muscle weakness and bone breakdown, which led to a condition called osteoporosis, in which bones are weakened and the risk of bone fractures or breaks is increased. Thyroid hormone extracts also made the heart work harder by increasing metabolism, which led to problems such as increased heart rate, palpitations, and irregular heartbeat. These problems were potentially life threatening: When the heart beats abnormally (or not at all), it is unable to pump blood and oxygen to the brain and body. Individuals die suddenly from this condition because the brain can only function for a few minutes without oxygen and nutrients.

Many people took thyroid drugs for weight loss before it was discovered that they could lead to serious health problems.

Thyroid hormones are still available, with a prescription, for patients with an underactive thyroid (hypothyroidism). These drugs are never given for weight loss.

DINITROPHENOL

Another drug that came in "under the radar"—that is, before FDA review or doctors' prescriptions were required—was dinitrophenol. Dinitrophenol, which was later discovered to be a respiratory poison, was introduced for weight loss in 1933. This drug increased metabolism to induce weight loss. Used alone, or with thyroid hormones, dinitrophenol produced rapid weight loss accompanied by symptoms of warmth, sweating, and fever. Approximately 100,000 people were treated with dinitrophenol before it was found to produce extremely dangerous side effects, including liver problems, vision impairment (from formation of cataracts), a weakening of the body's ability to fight infection, lung problems, and even death. Dinitrophenol was removed from the market in 1934, but not before many people became ill or died from its effects.

AMPHETAMINE-LIKE WEIGHT LOSS PRODUCTS
Amphetamine

Amphetamines, which were introduced in 1938, rapidly became the most widely used agents for the treatment of obesity in the United States. Amphetamine (Figure 4.1) is a stimulant that causes the release of the neurotransmitter norepinephrine in the brain, which leads to increased metabolism and increased energy expenditure, or burning of calories. Amphetamine is also an appetite suppressant. From the 1940s through the 1960s, individuals took "rainbow pills" for weight loss. These pills were called "rainbow pills" because of the number of drugs they contained: amphetamine, thyroid hormone, laxatives (to cause diarrhea and decrease food absorption in the gut), and diuretics (to increase urination

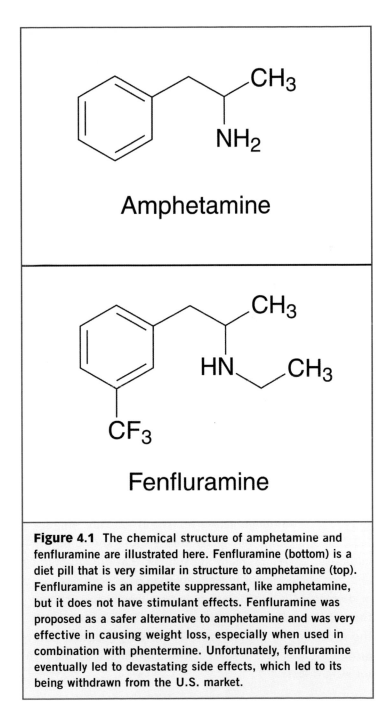

Figure 4.1 The chemical structure of amphetamine and fenfluramine are illustrated here. Fenfluramine (bottom) is a diet pill that is very similar in structure to amphetamine (top). Fenfluramine is an appetite suppressant, like amphetamine, but it does not have stimulant effects. Fenfluramine was proposed as a safer alternative to amphetamine and was very effective in causing weight loss, especially when used in combination with phentermine. Unfortunately, fenfluramine eventually led to devastating side effects, which led to its being withdrawn from the U.S. market.

and cause loss of water weight). Amphetamine, alone or in combination with other drugs, was very effective in causing weight loss but led to devastating side effects.

The side effects of amphetamine are related to its stimulant effects, especially at high doses and with long-term use. Side effects include irritability, insomnia, confusion, anxiety, paranoia, hallucinations, seizures, and aggressiveness. Amphetamines cause irreversible destruction of blood vessels in the brain, which can cause stroke—even in young people. These drugs also cause the potentially lethal side effects of increased heart rate, irregular heartbeat, and increased blood pressure.

Another problem with amphetamines is that they have a high potential for abuse. Amphetamine is very similar to the compound methamphetamine, which is known on the street today as "speed," "meth," or "crank." Both amphetamine and methamphetamine are "uppers," and are highly addictive. Besides causing weight loss, these drugs elevate a person's mood and cause euphoria, excitement, and ecstasy. People who experience these feelings tend to use the drugs more frequently, and at higher doses, to continue to experience this effect.

AMPHETAMINE

Amphetamine was the original stimulant used to induce weight loss. Although very effective at causing weight loss, amphetamine has many side effects and is highly addictive. Therefore, many substances that are structurally and funtionally similar to amphetamine have been developed or discovered in an attempt to induce weight loss without the negative effects of amphetamine. These drugs, with the exception of phentermine and diethylpropion, have proven to be unsafe and are not recommended by the FDA for weight loss.

Amphetamines are very effective for weight loss but their use is limited by serious side effects and the potential for abuse. Therefore, amphetamine is still FDA approved for other diseases but is no longer permitted for weight loss. Many drugs that are similar to amphetamine have been formulated in an attempt to promote weight loss without causing addiction and dangerous side effects.

MARY

Mary wanted to lose the weight she had gained during her pregnancy with her first child, who was now three years old. She hoped to lose the 30 pounds quickly, since she wanted to look her best when her husband returned in four months from active duty in World War II. Mary's sister told her all the movie stars were taking rainbow pills, which "worked like magic." At the corner drugstore, Mary bought a month's supply of rainbow pills, which came in four beautiful bottles. Within one week of taking these pills, Mary had lost five pounds. She was extremely excited that she could finally meet her weight loss goals. However, Mary began to feel nervous. She also experienced heart palpitations and dizziness when she stood up. She slept less and less. Before long, Mary began to feel that she could not get through the day without taking the pills. As the time of her husband's arrival drew near, she began to take more and more of her pills, since she was still 10 pounds short of her goal. One week before the day of her husband's return, Mary passed out at home. Smelling salts would not wake her and a doctor pronounced her dead one hour later.

The rainbow pills Mary had taken to lose weight caused her heart to race faster and faster, until eventually it simply stopped working.

Fenfluramine and Dexfenfluramine

Fenfluramine and dexfenfluramine were marketed under the brand names Redux® and Pondimin®, respectively. Fenfluramine and dexfenfluramine are chemically similar to amphetamine, but they work differently in the body. These drugs exert their effects by increasing the release of serotonin (a neurotransmitter) in the brain, leading to appetite suppression. Fenfluramine ("fen") and dexfenfluramine ("dexfen") were prescription appetite suppressants that had been approved by the FDA for the short-term management of obesity. A landmark study completed in 1992 showed that fenfluramine, when combined with the weight-loss drug phentermine, was very effective for weight loss over the short term. The study results were widely reported, and they led to a surge in popularity of fenfluramine and phentermine. This drug combination, called "fen-phen," was very effective and proved far more effective than either drug used alone.[5] The combination of dexfenfluramine and phentermine ("dexfen-phen") had similar effects on weight loss. The FDA never approved the use of these drugs together, however. The drugs, individually or together, were not intended to be used for longer than three months.

Initially, fen-phen was thought to be free of serious side effects. Short-term studies showed the main side effects to be tiredness and diarrhea, and these side effects went away as time passed and the body got used to the drugs. It was known that the "fen-phen" and "dexfen-phen" regimens led to rare cases of heart, lung, and nerve damage when used for a long time. Unfortunately, many doctors continued to prescribe these combinations for long-term use. This allowed patients who wanted to lose weight—often for cosmetic rather than health reasons—to do so and maintain the weight loss.

Many people stayed on the "fen-phen" or "dexfen-phen" regimens far longer than the recommended three months to continue or maintain their weight loss. Serious, life-threatening side effects became evident with long-term use of these combinations. Patients developed a lung disease called *primary pulmonary hypertension* (PPH), heart valve disease, and other conditions that were irreversible and in some cases life-threatening. PPH is a serious, permanent lung condition that can lead to breathing problems, heart failure, and death. A study investigating the link between fenfluramine and PPH concluded that patients using the diet drugs for longer than three months were 23 times more likely to develop PPH. These horrible effects were attributed mainly to fenfluramine and dexfenfluramine, and eventually the FDA banned these drugs from the market. Phentermine is still available for weight loss. It will be discussed in Chapter 5.

The most startling and damaging news regarding "fen-phen" and "dexfen-phen" came when the Mayo Clinic, in June 1997, reported 24 cases of heart valve damage in "fen-phen" users. Individuals in the study used "fen-phen" for an average of 12 months, well exceeding the recommended three months. Fenfluramine and dexfenfluramine caused leakage in the heart valves. The mitral and aortic valves, which control blood flow through part of the heart, were most affected. Valve leakage prevents the heart from pumping effectively. In five cases, patients required open heart valve surgery.

After many health problems and deaths, the FDA removed Pondimin and Redux from market. Since then, there have been 200 reported cases of primary pulmonary hypertension relating to "fen-phen" and "dexfen-phen." Of those cases, 40 have resulted in death. The FDA has received more than 100 reports of heart valve damage directly related to "fen-phen" or fenfluramine therapy; there are no reports from individuals taking phentermine alone for weight loss.

Phenylpropanolamine

Phenylpropanolamine is similar to amphetamine, but does not cause euphoria and does not have the same potential for abuse. Phenylpropanolamine was used as a cough and cold agent initially, since it relieves congestion associated with the common cold. Before long, people realized that it caused appetite suppression and that they were able to lose weight while taking it. In the 1940s, phenylpropanolamine became popular as a diet aid and stimulant. In 1951, the FDA enacted laws requiring people to have a doctor's prescription to obtain certain drugs; phenylpropanolamine, however, was not covered by these regulations.

ANGELA

Angela celebrated her engagement over Memorial Day weekend. The wedding would take place in the fall and Angela wanted to lose 25 pounds before buying her wedding gown. To help her lose weight, Angela's doctor prescribed a new diet-drug combination called "fen-phen." Angela never bought the gown.

About one month after beginning the "fen-phen" regimen, Angela became dizzy and short of breath. She stopped taking the drugs, but it was too late. In the hospital, Angela was diagnosed with primary pulmonary hypertension (PPH), a condition in which the blood pressure in the lungs rises dangerously high. Angela's PPH developed as a result of the "fen-phen" pills. The surgeon inserted a tube into Angela's chest and plugged it into a computerized box that would pump medicine into her heart. She was later released from the hospital. That same day, she died at home.

The doctors had done all they could, but Angela's lungs were too damaged by the "fen-phen" pills, and she suffocated.

Phenylropanolamine was initially believed to have a very low risk of side effects, and the FDA allowed it to be available over the counter, without a prescription. After some time, phenylpropanolamine became the active ingredient in many nonprescription diet pills, such as Acutrim®, Dexatrim®, and Protrim. Early studies demonstrated that the drug's main side effect was an increase in energy that sometimes led to insomnia or agitation.

Phenylpropanolamine works by increasing dopamine and norepinephrine in the feeding center of the brain, which causes appetite suppression. Beginning in the 1970s, the FDA began to gather reports of individuals experiencing hemorrhagic stroke, a life-threatening bleeding in the brain or the tissue surrounding the brain, that was related to phenylpropanolamine's stimulant effects. These strokes generally occurred in young women and were suspected of being a result of very high blood pressure caused by phenylpropanolamine use.

In 2000, a report from Yale University determined that use of phenylprolamine-containing appetite suppressants made individuals 16 times more likely to have a hemorrhagic stroke.[6] Phenylpropanolamine had also been linked to heart attacks and high blood pressure in many patients. Therefore, in November 2000, the FDA asked pharmaceutical manufacturers to stop marketing products containing phenylpropanolamine. Many of the products originally containing phenylpropano-lamine are still legally available, but have been reformulated with a different active ingredient and no longer contain phenylpropanolamine.

Ephedra

Ephedra, also known as Ma-Huang, is a central nervous system stimulant that is similar to amphetamine. Ephedra alkaloids (a material found in plants) with the active ingredient ephedrine have been used for medicinal purposes in China for

STEVE BECHLER

Steve Bechler (Figure 4.2) was a 23-year-old pitcher for the Baltimore Orioles who, at 6'2" and 239 pounds, had constantly struggled with his weight. On Monday, February 17, 2004—just 27 days after Bechler had joined the team at its spring training facility in Fort Lauderdale, Florida—he died of heatstroke during a morning workout. The temperature outside was only 81°F. Although similar incidents had happened in professional and college football, this was the first report of a major league baseball player dying of heatstroke. What caused this horrible event? A bottle of Xenadrine™, a product containing ephedra, was found in Bechler's pocket. He had been taking the product three times a day to increase his energy and assist with weight loss. Medical examiners agreed that the ephedra contributed to Bechler's death by increasing his metabolism. Bechler's body temperature was 108°F when he died, which caused several of his internal organs to fail.

Steve Bechler was denied a successful career and would never get to see his first child, which he and his wife, Kylie, were expecting at the time of his death.

generations. Ephedra acts like the body's natural adrenaline and is used to boost energy levels and induce weight loss. Ephedra is an appetite suppressant and increases metabolism, especially when combined with caffeine. Ephedra was marketed as a dietary supplement, not a drug, and therefore, the FDA had little control over it prior to its being released (although the FDA does have the ability to pull a supplement from the market if that supplement has been proven unsafe.) Manufacturers did not have to prove it was safe or effective before it was

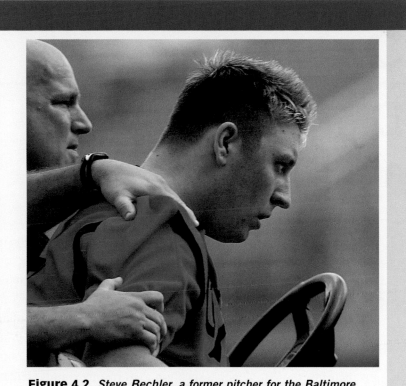

Figure 4.2 *Steve Bechler, a former pitcher for the Baltimore Orioles, died after taking a weight loss supplement containing ephedra. Here he is being taken off the playing field during training camp, when he began to suffer from heat exhaustion, a side effect of ephedra-based drugs.*

marketed. Ephedra, found in many dietary supplements, was a popular stimulant and weight loss pill for years.

Ephedra, like amphetamine, raises heart rate and blood pressure. It was shown to increase the risk of heart attack, seizure, stroke, and sudden death. In February 2004, the FDA finally had enough information to prove ephedra was unsafe and was able to remove it from the U.S. market.

5

Diet Pills
and the FDA

Each year, millions of Americans resolve to lose weight—it is one of
the most common New Year's resolutions. Many people start off
with great intentions, but within months, weeks, or even days, most
of them give up and return to their usual habits. If they work to
lose weight, the possibility exists that they might end up regaining
any weight they lost. Americans spend up to $30 billion each year on
various methods of weight loss, and often see little improvement
for their investment. Money is spent on gym memberships, exercise
equipment, and weight loss supplements.[7] For many morbidly
obese people, the only way they can get on the road to successful
weight loss is though the use of drugs or other medical interventions.

Over the years, experts' rationale for incorporating obesity drugs
into established guidelines has changed. There are several reasons for
this. Top among these are that experts realize that obesity and overweight are major health problems, and can develop into lifelong
diseases. These factors indicate that obesity is a chronic (long-term)
disease (Figure 5.1). Children who are obese often remain obese or overweight as adults. This chapter focuses on the use, risks, and benefits
of prescription drugs that are approved by the FDA for weight loss.

QUALIFYING FOR DRUG THERAPY
For an overweight or obese person to qualify for drug therapy, he or
she must meet certain criteria. These are:

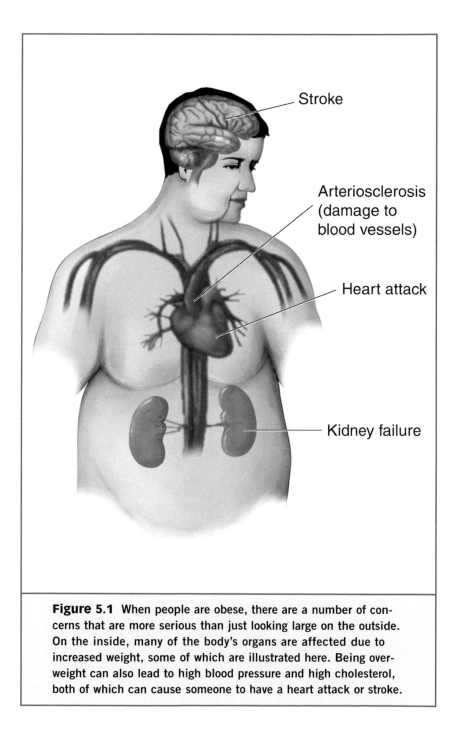

Stroke

Arteriosclerosis
(damage to
blood vessels)

Heart attack

Kidney failure

Figure 5.1 When people are obese, there are a number of concerns that are more serious than just looking large on the outside.
On the inside, many of the body's organs are affected due to
increased weight, some of which are illustrated here. Being overweight can also lead to high blood pressure and high cholesterol,
both of which can cause someone to have a heart attack or stroke.

1. The patient must have a BMI greater than 30 kg/m^2.

   OR

2. The patient must have a BMI greater than 27 kg/m^2
   and risk factors for:

   a. High blood pressure;

   b. High levels of cholesterol in the blood.

   OR

3. The patient must have a waist circumference greater
   than 35 inches (89 cm) for women or 40 inches
   (102 cm) for men, and the risk factors stated above.

It is important to realize that people who qualify for drug therapy do so based on health considerations and risk factors, not simply because they want to improve their appearance. Drug therapy is not undertaken for cosmetic reasons and should never be regarded as a shortcut or "springboard" to weight loss. Healthy diet and exercise are the keys to weight loss.

Diet drugs alone will not produce weight loss. A patient must be engaged in an appropriate weight loss program that includes regular exercise. If someone wishes to lose weight over the long term, he or she must be committed to staying on his or her weight loss program. Diet drugs are not the "be all, end all" of weight loss.

HOW THE FDA APPROVES DRUGS

The FDA's approval process for new prescription drugs is extensive. It can take over ten years for a drug to reach the market. Before receiving FDA approval, a new drug must be studied extensively. The process begins with the discovery or development of a new substance that can be used for medicinal purposes. The potential drug is first studied in a laboratory, then in animals. It is then studied in healthy adults to see what effects it produces and to determine how it works in the body. In the next phase of studies, the drug is given to a large number of people who are "sick," to see if the drug is effective.

If the drug passes through these rounds of testing, it is subjected to a thorough review by an FDA advisory committee, which determines from all of the information the company submits whether or not the drug works. Considerable emphasis is also put on the safety of this new drug. If the drug passes the FDA's review, it can be put on the market. The result of this extensive review process is, ideally, a new, effective, safe drug that can help a person combat a disease (such as obesity) that can result in very serious outcomes.

DRUGS APPROVED BY THE FDA FOR WEIGHT LOSS

Drugs approved for use in weight loss programs can be broken down into the following categories.

1. Anorexiants (drugs that work on chemicals in the brain)

   a. Amphetamines

      1. Benzphetamine (Didrex®)

      2. Diethylpriopion (Tenuate®; Tenuate Dospan®)

      3. Methamphetamine (Desoxyn®)

      4. Phentermine (Adipex®; Adipex®-P or Ionamin®)

   b. Sibutramine (Meridia®)

2. Lipase Inhibitors (drugs that prevent fat from being absorbed into the bloodstream)

   a. Orlistat

Drugs that work in the brain are considered appetite suppressants. Amphetamines are approved for use in treating other diseases; their use as a weight loss drug is considered "off label," or not approved. Doctors often prescribe drugs for "off-label" use, meaning that the drug is used at a different dose, for a longer time, or for a different medical condition than was approved by the FDA. Off-label prescribing is a common, and legal, practice.

Amphetamines, which have appetite-suppressing effects, are approved by the FDA for weight loss, but only for short-term use (12 weeks or less). Only a handful of studies have evaluated their use for periods longer than six months. Scientists do not fully understand how amphetamines and amphetamine-like drugs work. It is believed that these drugs cause the release of norepinephrine and dopamine, two chemical messengers that control hunger, in the brain. In addition, it is thought that amphetamines decrease the sharpness of a person's senses of smell and taste, which ultimately results in appetite-suppressing properties.

Another benefit of amphetamines is that they allow someone who is obese or overweight the opportunity and time to learn proper weight loss techniques, such as diet and exercise. Because they are addictive, amphetamines are not often recommended for use in weight loss. Amphetamines and amphetamine-like drugs only bring about a very small amount of weight loss (3–8% decrease in weight when compared to placebo). So, since amphetamines are addictive and not very effective for long-term weight control, they are not recommended for weight loss.

Amphetamines and amphetamine-like drugs only bring about a very small amount of weight loss. The usual weight loss that occurs is only 5 to 10 pounds. Often, the weight loss effects only last for a few weeks. The way these drugs help induce weight loss is by providing the patient the time and opportunity he or she needs to learn proper weight loss techniques.

BENZPHETAMINE (DIDREX®) AND METHAMPHETAMINE (DESOXYN®)

Benzphetamine and methamphetamine are similar to

amphetamine both structurally and functionally. They work by stimulating nerves in the brain, which increases heart rate and blood pressure while decreasing appetite. Benzphetamine is prescribed to be taken once a day 30 to 60 minutes before breakfast. Methamphetamine is given in 5-mg doses 30 minutes before each meal. It is important not to increase the dose or take the drug more often then the doctor says. Usually, these drugs are taken for 8 to 12 weeks. An illegal form of methamphetamine called "crank" is made in underground laboratories from over-the-counter drugs such as Sudafed® and sold as a drug of abuse. Often, "crank" contains many other illegal compounds that work to produce psychological effects.

People who are obese, and who have diabetes, often find they initially cannot control their blood sugar well. Therefore, these patients must increase the number of times each day they monitor their blood sugar. Benzphetamine, out of the entire amphetamine class, causes less stimulant activity; this quality could make it more attractive to doctors. But tolerance (the body's ability to resist the effects of the drug) can develop quickly and adequate weight loss has not been observed beyond six months.

DIETHYLPROPION (TENUATE®; TENUATE DOSPAN®)

Diethylpropion is also similar to amphetamine in both structure and function. This drug is available in an immediate-release form (which must be taken more often during the day) and as a controlled-release preparation that is only taken once a day. The dose of this drug is usually 25 mg taken three times a day before meals; the controlled-release product is taken 75 mg mid-morning. The last dose of diethylpropion should be taken four to six hours before bedtime. Studies have shown that people taking diethylpropion achieve a weight loss of 17.4 to 19.1 pounds at six to 12 months. This is in comparison to people who took a sugar pill and lost no weight.

PHENTERMINE (ADIPEX®; ADIPEX®-P OR IONAMIN®)

Phentermine (Figure 5.2) is similar to amphetamine both structurally and functionally, but has less potential for abuse. It is available in both an immediate-release and sustained-release form. The dose is 30 mg once a day in the morning. Some doctors prescribe smaller doses to be taken with every meal. Phentermine has been found to be effective for weight loss, but only when used along with diet, exercise, and other behaviors, such as simply setting up a weight goal or rewarding weight loss. Researchers have found that people may not need phentermine for long periods of time, but only from time to time. Some people who take phentermine end up regaining weight that they lost, even while still taking the drug, and often stop using it because they feel it is not working.

SIDE EFFECTS OF AMPHETAMINES

The largest drawback to the use of amphetamines is the often severe side effects that can occur. All amphetamines can cause nervousness, dry mouth, insomnia, anxiety, elevated heart rate, high blood pressure, and heart palpitations. Another side effect of amphetamines is artificially elevated feelings of self-confidence. Abusers of amphetamines have a false sense of well-being; they feel like they are invincible and could "conquer the world."

Another major drawback of amphetamines and amphetamine-like drugs is that because their appetite-suppressive effects do not last long, their weight loss effects wear off after a short time. This is why physicians prescribe some of them to be used for only a few days at a time, then put the patient on a "drug holiday" for the next few days. This routine allows for the effective use of these drugs over a longer period of time. There are only a few agents approved for use in treating obesity. The fact that these agents are not prescribed frequently reflects the point that they can be potentially dangerous to use.

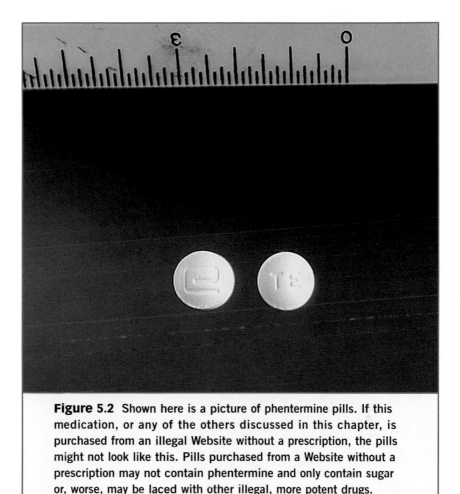

Figure 5.2 Shown here is a picture of phentermine pills. If this medication, or any of the others discussed in this chapter, is purchased from an illegal Website without a prescription, the pills might not look like this. Pills purchased from a Website without a prescription may not contain phentermine and only contain sugar or, worse, may be laced with other illegal, more potent drugs.

In addition to all of the side effects they can cause, another problem with amphetamines is that people can rapidly develop an addiction to them. The addiction starts because these agents are like speed, an illegal drug that "revs up" the body. It also has the ability to induce a feeling of euphoria, which is what makes the drug so appealing and addictive. Speed makes the heart beat faster, which has the effect of keeping the body moving even when it is extremely fatigued. Amphetamines offer the appealing benefit of allowing a person to sleep less and accomplish more. However, amphetamine addiction does produce problems in the body. Signs of addiction include:

- An uncontrollable desire to continue taking the drug longer than the doctor recommends

- Hallucinations

- A need to increase the dose (tolerance) to feel the same effects

- Sleeplessness

- Irritability

- Personality changes

- Psychosis, often clinically indistinguishable from schizophrenia (a mental disorder)—this is the most serious sign of amphetamine addiction.

When a person who is addicted to amphetamines suddenly stops taking the drug, he or she usually experiences unpleasant withdrawal symptoms, including:

- Sleepiness

- Vomiting

- Stomach cramps

- Trembling.

When a person taking amphetamines stops taking them, his or her body may need to adjust. How long these withdrawal symptoms last depends on how long and how often the drug was taken. Often, a person will experience feelings of being extremely tired, weak, and easily confused—these feelings go away in time.

SIBUTRAMINE (MERIDIA®)

Sibutramine is approved by the FDA for long-term management of weight loss; it can be used for approximately one year.

Sibutramine is a noradrenergic and serotonergic agent, which means that it works by suppressing the neurotransmitters in the brain that control appetite, and by increasing the rate at which food is broken down. Studies have shown that patients taking sibutramine achieve an average weight loss of 17.6 pounds (8 kg) to 19.8 pounds (9 kg), although some patients have been able to lose more.

The starting dose of sibutramine is usually 10 to 15 mg once a day. The drawback of this drug is that, as with all medications used to treat obesity, the lost weight eventually reappears unless the patient continues to engage in healthy eating habits and an exercise program.

One study of people who used sibutramine for two years (although the FDA only approved one year of use) showed one possibly positive effect of this drug: continued weight maintenance. In this study, over 80% of people who took sibutramine for two years kept their weight constant. Along with the maintained weight loss, researchers also found that patients were able to decrease the lipid (fat) in their bloodstream, which has beneficial effects on the health of the heart.

Sibutramine use also carries the risk of side effects, which include elevated blood pressure, increased heart rate, dry mouth, nausea, and dizziness. Abuse of sibutramine can cause dilated pupils, excessive bleeding or bruising, tremor, and anxiety. As with all prescription drugs, it is essential to use sibutramine according a doctor's instructions. The alternative is the possibility of unpleasant side effects and dangerous outcomes.

ORLISTAT (XENICAL®)

The last class of weight-loss drugs approved by the FDA is lipase inhibitors. Drugs in this category prevent the body from absorbing fat into the bloodstream, which creates conditions that make it easier for weight loss to occur. Clinical studies have shown that lipase inhibitors produce a dose-dependent decrease of weight (meaning that at low doses, a person sees less weight loss than would be seen at higher doses). Most patients who take these drugs achieve a loss of 6.6 pounds (3 kg) to 8.8 pounds (4 kg). The usual dose of these drugs is 120 mg three times a day. Patients must be sure to take a multivitamin each day—it has been found that in addition to decreasing the amount of fat ingested with each meal, lipase inhibitors also block the absorption of essential vitamins in food.

One study undertaken to assess lipase inhibitors in overweight, diabetic patients concluded that these patients not only achieved significant weight loss but were also better able to control their blood sugar. Other studies have shown that patients who were at high risk for developing diabetes did not do so when taking orlistat; in these patients, excess weight was the cause of developing diabetes.

The side effects of orlistat are extremely unpleasant. Patients may experience abdominal pain, gas, and discomfort when taking this drug; the abdominal problems that occur are even more intense after the patient eats a high-fat meal. Since orlistat is a lipase inhibitor, it prevents fat from being absorbed by the body. Thus, the fat in food comes out of the body in the stool, causing these side effects:

- Soft stools

- Abdominal pain

- Flatulence

- The sudden need to go to the bathroom

- Not being able stop a bowel movement from happening

- Oily discharge.

Often, these effects make people stop taking lipase inhibitors almost as soon as they start it. Most patients are unwilling or unable to endure the side effects. Patients soon realize that these effects become less intense when they change their diet and eat foods that are lower in fat.

There is not a significant abuse potential with lipase inhibitors. If abuse occurs, the patient experiences even more severe forms of the drug's already unpleasant side effects, and

FRANK

Frank is 44 years old, 5 feet 8 inches tall, and weighs 190 lbs. His BMI is 27 and, thus, he is considered overweight. Frank is taking a prescription medicine to help manage his diabetes. He also has high blood pressure. His doctor has told him that he must lower his weight to get his diabetes and high blood pressure under control.

He has tried on his own to lose weight. He started going to Weight Watchers™ and is walking more. In spite of this, he is not losing any weight. His doctor told him about a prescription medication called Xenical®, which may help him lose weight. Xenical does not interact with any of the medications he is taking right now.

Frank decided that he would try taking this medicine. Although plagued with multiple side effects that affected mainly his bowels, he lost weight. He knew that if he ate fewer fatty foods, the digestive side effects would lessen. He did this and stuck with the medication. He has lost 15 pounds and would like to lose more. Frank has already seen a change in his blood pressure, and his diabetes medicine dosage is lower.

Frank is motivated and wants to lose weight. He has lost weight and does not want to look back on the days when he was overweight. He wants to continue to lose and maintain his weight loss, not only for cosmetic reasons, but because he realizes the negative health effects of being overweight.

thus people often avoid taking the drug if it is not necessary, or avoid taking more of it than prescribed.

GUIDELINES FOR USE OF WEIGHT CONTROL DRUGS

The National Institutes of Health (NIH) has developed a list of guidelines that should be used when a patient is prescribed a weight loss drug. If a patient does not meet all criteria for drug therapy, then diet and exercise should be used instead. Weight loss drugs come with many side effects and contraindications (reasons why the drug should not be used), and they can be addicting and lethal. The NIH guidelines recommend that:

1. All individuals begin with diet modification and exercise.

2. If diet changes do not bring about weight loss (10% of initial body weight or 1 pound (0.5 kg) per week), drug therapy may be started.

3. If the patient does not lose 4.4 pounds (2 kg) in the first four weeks of drug treatment, drug therapy might have to be changed or the dose increased when possible.

There is an increasing interest in weight loss drugs among doctors and consumers. Because of adverse effects that may occur, it is important for doctors and patients to proceed with drug therapy very cautiously. Drug therapy for overweight and obesity is only based on a small number of clinical trials. Weight loss drugs should only be used as part of a program that includes diet and physical activity. The patient must be taught to set weight goals that he or she can achieve and give him- or herself rewards for weight loss. Obviously, once a weight loss drug is no longer being taken, diet and exercise are the only ways that weight can be lost. The manufacturers of drugs to treat obesity must continue to work toward developing safer and more effective products.

6

Dietary Supplements for Weight Loss

Dietary supplements are popular products for weight loss. These products are often promoted with elaborate advertising campaigns, often using celebrity endorsements (Figure 6.1) that promise consumers they will lose weight and feel wonderful. Many people believe that since these products are "natural," they are safe. The reality is that "natural" means we do not always know exactly what active ingredients are contained in a product. "Natural" does not equal safe. Still, many Americans purchase these products at health-food stores, pharmacies, and over the Internet, hoping to achieve the risk-free, miraculous weight-loss results promised in advertisements. Unfortunately, many of these Americans end up having reason to regret that decision.

What defines a dietary supplement versus a drug? As defined by Congress in the Dietary Supplement Health and Education Act (which became law in 1994), a dietary supplement is a product (other than tobacco) that:

- is intended to supplement the diet;
- contains one or more dietary ingredients (including vitamins, minerals, herbs or other botanicals, amino acids, and other substances);
- is intended to be taken by mouth as a pill, capsule, tablet, or liquid; and
- is labeled on the front panel as being a dietary supplement.

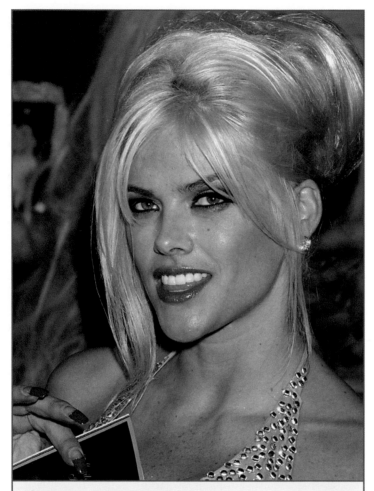

Figure 6.1 Anna Nicole Smith, a famous actress and model, reports that she used the dietary supplement TrimSpa™ to achieve her recent weight loss. Advertisements like these encourage consumers to believe they will achieve miraculous weight loss results, i.e., look like a runway model, if they use this product. These advertisements never even hint at the potential side effects associated with this diet pill.

One distinction between drugs and dietary supplements is how they are regulated by the FDA. Unlike for drugs, manufacturers do not have to provide FDA with evidence that dietary supplements are effective or safe before the products are marketed; however, they are not permitted to continue marketing unsafe or ineffective products. Once a dietary supplement reaches the market, the FDA must prove that the product is not safe in order to restrict its use or remove it from the market. In contrast, for drugs, the burden of proof is on the manufacturers to convincingly establish a drug's safety and efficacy before receiving FDA approval and being allowed to bring the drug to market.

Unlike with drugs, manufacturers of dietary supplements do not have to disclose potential side effects of their products to consumers. The label of the supplement may contain a cautionary statement, but the lack of such a statement does not mean that no adverse effects are associated with the product. Dietary supplements may also interfere with the activity of other medicines (drugs or other supplements) an individual is taking. Also unlike with drugs, the manufacturer is not required to disclose these interactions to the consumer.

Besides safety and effectiveness, the FDA does not regulate manufacturing processes for dietary supplements as strictly as it does for drugs. There are no FDA regulations for dietary supplements that correspond to the Good Manufacturing Practices (GMPs) standard the agency applies to pharmaceutical manufacturers. The only pre-marketing regulation of dietary supplements performed by the FDA occurs in cases where a new dietary ingredient is developed. The FDA reviews the product for safety, but the manufacturer does not have to provide the FDA with proof that the product is effective before or after it markets it. Standardization is a process that manufacturers may use to ensure that there is a consistency of quality between batches of product; however, U.S. dietary supplements manufacturers are not held to any federal standardization requirements. In fact, no legal or regulatory definition exists in the United States for standardization as it applies to dietary supplements. Therefore, two bottles of the same product may contain completely different amounts of active ingredient, which means you cannot be sure that the product you purchase actually contains the ingredients listed on the label.

WITHDRAWAL OF EPHEDRA

Products containing ephedra were used extensively by the American public for weight loss and to enhance athletic performance. Ephedra, a stimulant similar to amphetamine, increases blood pressure and heart rate after only one dose, significantly increasing a person's risk of heart attack, stroke, and death. Because ephedra is a dietary supplement, the FDA did not review its safety or efficacy before it became available to the American public. According to law, the FDA could only prohibit the sale of the dietary supplement if it was proven to present a significant or unreasonable risk of injury.

In February 2004, the FDA withdrew ephedra, one of the most popular dietary supplements, from the market because it finally had enough information to prove that ephedra presented an unreasonable risk of illness or injury under the conditions of use recommended on the product labeling. This withdrawal did not happen until many people suffered from the terrible potential side effects of this supplement (see Chapter 4).

The ephedra case illustrates an important point about dietary supplements, perhaps best expressed in the Latin expression *caveat emptor*, or, literally, "let the buyer beware." Because the FDA does not regulate dietary supplements as strictly as it regulates drugs, consumers must educate themselves and make informed decisions when deciding to consume dietary supplements for weight loss. It can never be assumed that these products are safe because they are natural. Talk with your doctor or pharmacist before you take any supplement. Some supplements may interact with prescription or over-the-counter medications, possibly decreasing the effectiveness of your medications. They might also complicate an existing condition, or even cause one, such as high blood pressure.

Thousands of dietary supplements are marketed for the purpose of weight loss. It would be impossible to cover each of these individual products in this chapter. Instead, this chapter will familiarize you with common ingredients found in many dietary supplements. You are encouraged to review ingredients in common dietary supplements for weight loss to understand the potential positive and negative effects of these products.

STIMULANTS

With the withdrawal of ephedra from the U.S. market, companies producing dietary supplements for weight loss have replaced ephedra with other stimulants to induce weight loss. Many of these stimulants contain caffeine or are very similar to caffeine. Caffeine and related substances suppress appetite and cause increased metabolism, thus causing the body to burn more calories. The increase in metabolism causes the body to produce more heat (thermogenesis). Most of these agents are probably safe in very low doses. However, side effects increase when these products are taken in high doses or in combination with other stimulants. Especially in high doses, stimulants like caffeine have the potential to cause nervousness, insomnia, increased heart rate, high blood pressure, abnormal heartbeat, and palpitations. Caffeine also causes psychological dependence and can cause withdrawal symptoms if discontinued abruptly. The increase in metabolism caused by these agents also makes body organs, especially the heart, work harder, which can lead to side effects over the long term. Supplements that contain stimulants should be avoided by women who are pregnant or breastfeeding and by individuals with underlying heart disease or high blood pressure. Many of these supplements have not been well studied and may have other serious side effects that are unknown at this time.

Guarana

Guarana, a stimulant very similar to caffeine, grows as a shrub in the Amazon (Figure 6.2). Guarana was initially made into a beverage by the Maue Indians in the Amazon Basin as a daily tonic and stimulant, much like coffee. In fact, 100 mg of guarana is approximately equivalent to the caffeine contained in one cup of black coffee. The Maue Indians believed guarana warded off headaches, relieved cramps and fevers, and was an aphrodisiac (a substance that stimulates sexual feelings). Today, guarana is still a popular stimulant beverage, especially in Brazil. Guarana is currently marketed in the United States, Canada, and European countries as a stimulant, appetite suppressant, smoking cessation aid, pain reliever, aphrodisiac, and as a flavoring for commercial soft drinks.

Guarana contains tetra methylxanthine, a compound almost identical to caffeine and other stimulants such as theophylline (which has been isolated and sold as a drug and which can be toxic when consumed in high doses), theobromine, and saponins. Although not well documented, the side effects of guarana are similar to those of other stimulants.

Bitter Orange

Bitter orange is an extract of the fruit and peel of the Seville orange and is found in foods such as orange marmalade. It is taken from the plant *Citrus aurantium* and is also called Zhi Shi by Chinese herbalists. Although safe in the tiny amounts found in food, bitter orange has yet to be proven safe in the larger quantities used in supplements. Bitter orange is supposed to increase metabolism, suppress appetite, and reduce the conversion of carbohydrates to fat. Bitter orange contains the active ingredient synephrine, a stimulant that is very similar to ephedrine. Bitter orange also contains the stimulants tyramine and octopamine.

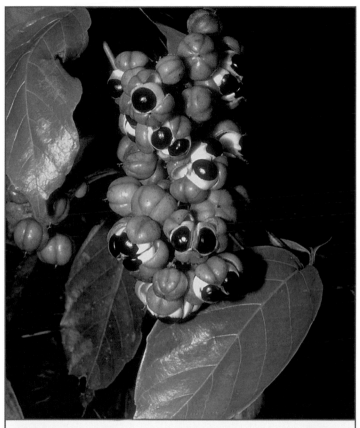

Figure 6.2 Guarana, shown here, grows as a shrub in the Amazon. The Maue Indians initially made this herb into a beverage that they used as a stimulant to keep them attentive on hunting trips. The Maue Indians also believed guarana had medicinal uses. Today, guarana is still a popular stimulant beverage, especially in Brazil, and is used in dietary supplements to help people lose weight.

Yerba Mate

Yerba Mate (*Ilex paraguariensis*) is a small tree native to the subtropical highlands of Brazil, Paraguay, Uruguay, and Argentina. This evergreen member of the holly family was introduced to colonizing and modern civilizations by the Guarani Indians of Paraguay and Uruguay.

A drink of the same name (Figure 6.3) is brewed from the dried leaves and stemlets of this perennial (a tree that thrives all year long). Yerba Mate is known as the national drink of these countries, and is consumed by millions of South Americans as an alternative to coffee. This stimulating herbal beverage is purported to have the unique ability to wake up the mind without the nervousness and jitters associated with coffee. In South America, the morning and afternoon beverage of choice is Yerba Mate. In fact, "mate bars" are as prevalent in South American countries as coffeehouses are here in the United States. According to a survey, Yerba Mate is consumed by 92% of households in Argentina.

Kola Nut

Kola nut, also known as cola nut, cola, and African kola nut, is the seed kernel of a several large trees native to Africa. It is extremely popular in the tropics as a caffeine-containing stimulant. Historically, it was believed to help hunters endure fatigue when food was not available. Today, kola nut is a stimulant and is believed to be an appetite suppressant, anti-depressant, diuretic (water pill), and astringent (a material that causes body tissues to tighten).

Green Tea Extract

Green tea has been used for generations in China as medicine to treat headaches, body aches, and poor digestion and to improve well-being and life expectancy. Ingredients in green tea include antioxidants, bioflavonoids, and caffeine. Green tea is probably safe in low doses, as it is consumed daily in many Asian cultures without reported side effects.

APPETITE SUPPRESSANTS

These agents are supposed to suppress appetite in various ways. Known active ingredients in these supplements are listed on the package; however, other, unknown active compounds may be

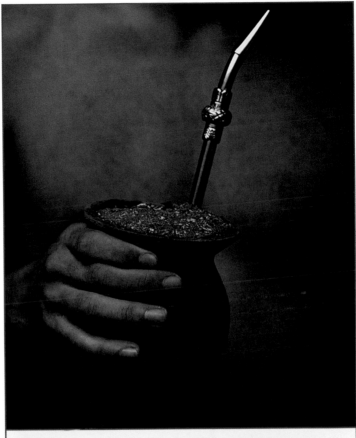

Figure 6.3 Yerba Mate is a small tree that grows in South America. Yerba Mate tea, made from the dried leaves and stemlets of the Yerba Mate tree, is a popular stimulant drink in South America. Yerba Mate is also used in many diet pills.

present in these herbal products. Similarly, whereas these products generally describe known side effects, other side effects may become evident with increased use of these supplements.

Hoodia gordonii

Hoodia gordonii was discovered and used by the San tribe, one of South Africa's oldest native peoples, since prehistoric times. The cactus *Hoodia gordonii* is a small, flowering cactus. Historically, people chewed the bitter stems of the cactus twice a day to stave off hunger and thirst during long hunting trips. The supplement made from *Hoodia* is believed to work in the brain to increase the feeling of satiety (fullness). This supplement was also believed to increase energy, so it may have some stimulant properties. Scientists have isolated an active ingredient in *Hoodia* that they have named P57. Safety and effectiveness of this ingredient are now being studied in scientific trials. If P57 proves to be safe and effective for weight loss, it will be formulated into a drug.

Hydroxycitric Acid

Hydroxycitric acid (HCA) is found in the fruit and rind of the mangosteen oil tree plant (*Garcinia campogia*). This tropical plant, native to India, bears yellowish pumpkin-shaped fruit (Figure 6.4). In animal studies, HCA was shown to decrease the body's conversion of calories to body fat and suppress appetite by increasing the use of the glycogen (sugar stores) for energy. These effects have not been consistently proven in human research. HCA is also reported to lower cholesterol; this claim has also not been proven. Few adverse effects have been reported with this agent, but those that have been seen include upset stomach and congestion (or "cold" symptoms).

Glucomannan

Glucomannan is a water-soluble (capable of being dissolved in water) dietary fiber derived from konjac root (*Amorphophallus konjac*). Like other forms of dietary fiber, glucomannan is considered a "bulk-forming laxative" and is used to treat constipation. Glucomannan may also help lower cholesterol and manage diabetes, although more trials are needed to prove these claims. Glucomannan may help with weight loss by occupying space in the stomach and making a person feel full, thus suppressing appetite. There are conflicting

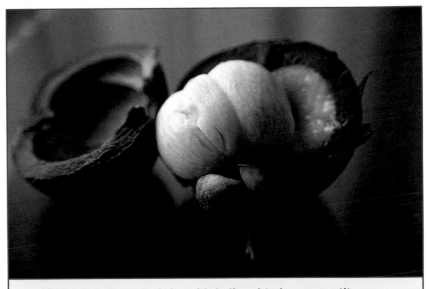

Figure 6.4 Hydroxycitric acid, believed to be an appetite suppressant, is found in the fruit and rind of the mangosteen oil tree plant. This tropical plant, native to India, bears yellowish pumpkin-shaped fruit (shown here). Hydroxycitric acid is found in many dietary supplements to aid in weight loss.

study results regarding the effectiveness of glucomannan for weight loss.

The main side effects of glucomannan include flatulence and stomach discomfort. Glucomannan may also expand in the esophagus (swallowing tube) and cause blockage if it is not taken with plenty of water. It can also interact with other medicines; it should be taken separately from other medicines by at least a couple of hours.

OTHER DIETARY SUPPLEMENTS FOR WEIGHT LOSS
Dehydroepiandosterone (DHEA)

DHEA is an adrenal hormone that is a precursor to the sex hormones testosterone and estrogen, as well as other hormones. DHEA is reported to increase testosterone and decrease total body fat, and also to have anabolic and anti-aging effects. The anabolic effects are of particular importance. Abuses of DHEA have the effect of a temporary increase in muscle size, an effect that many athletes desire. DHEA is banned by the International Olympic Committee (IOC) and the National Collegiate Athletic Association (NCAA) because of its similarity to anabolic steroids. Side effects of DHEA include acne, body hair growth, liver enlargement, and aggressiveness. This supplement should never be used during pregnancy, as it may be dangerous to the fetus. DHEA can have serious, life-threatening side effects with extended use and has raised concerns in the medical community. High doses of DHEA may increase the risk of prostate cancer, breast cancer, and other hormone-sensitive cancers.

JEFF

Jeff joined the football team his freshman year of college and immediately felt the pressure to lose body fat and get stronger before the season was under way. He was worried that, since he had not worked out during the summer like most of the other guys, he would never be selected to play first-string defensive back. One of the players told Jeff about a dietary supplement containing DHEA that could enhance muscle-building. Jeff assumed it would be safe, since it was not a drug and the bottle reported no side effects. Jeff took the supplement and he did begin to gain muscle and lose body fat. However, he developed severe acne and a sudden surge in the growth of body hair. He also began to develop fits of rage and was unable to control his temper. This was very unlike Jeff, who had never had a bad temper in the past.

Eventually, Jeff was asked to leave the football team, after a fistfight with a teammate sent the teammate to the hospital. Upon examination by a therapist, DHEA was implicated as the reason for Jeff's behavior.

Chromium

Chromium is a trace mineral that is necessary to process carbohydrates and fats, as well as to help cells respond properly to insulin—an especially important function for people with diabetes. Chromium, in its safest form, can be found in whole grains, seafood, green beans, peanut butter, and potatoes. As a dietary supplement, chromium is available in several forms, including chromium picolinate, chromium chloride, chromium nicotinate, and high-chromium yeast.

The weight-loss effects of chromium have not been proven. Chromium may be unsafe in high doses, especially when combined with picolinate. Specifically, chromium picolinate may cause headaches and mood disturbances. High doses may lead to blood and disorders of the liver and kidney, and may increase the risk of cancer.

Guggul

Guggul, also called guggulipid, is an extract from the gum resin of the Guggul tree, *Commiphora mukul,* a small bush native to India and Pakistan. This agent has been used in Indian tribal medicine for over 2,000 years to treat various ailments. Recently, guggul has been used as a dietary supplement to treat obesity, high cholesterol, and arthritis. Guggulsterones are the known active ingredient in guggul. Guggulsterones may function as a weight loss agent by increasing production of T_3, the most potent thyroid hormone, in the body. This increases metabolism and causes increased burning of calories. As discussed in Chapter 4, a long-term increase of thyroid hormones in the body leads to serious negative side effects including bone and muscle breakdown and heart problems.

BEING AN INFORMED CONSUMER

Now that you know more about some common ingredients found in dietary supplements for weight loss, you should make sure you read the ingredients on any supplements you may consider taking. If you find ingredients that have not been mentioned in this chapter, use books or credible information on the Internet to educate yourself about their risks and benefits. Dietary supplements are not strictly regulated for safety or effectiveness at this time, and there may be little to no strong evidence to support their use. This leaves the decision-making squarely up to you, the consumer. Have the manufacturer's claims about effectiveness been scientifically proven? Has the product's safety been tested? These are among the many considerations consumers must research and decide for themselves.

7

Diet Pill Abuse

This book has examined how diet pills work and which herbal and prescription products are most commonly used for weight loss. Disorders such as anorexia, bulimia, and body dysmorphic syndrome may lead someone to abuse both over-the-counter and prescription diet pills. There are health and legal ramifications of diet pill abuse that are ignored or not even realized when abuse is taking place.

STATISTICS REGARDING EATING DISORDERS

Eating disorders can be broken down into four categories: anorexia, bulimia, binge eating, and other disorders (such as body dysmorphic syndrome). Approximately 1% of female adolescents have anorexia; the mortality rate for anorexia in this age and gender group is higher than for any other psychological disorder, including depression. People with anorexia have different ages of onset of this disease. Thirty-three percent of anorexia patients develop (show signs of) anorexia when they are 11–15 years old; 43% of anorexia sufferers show signs of anorexia when they are 16–20 years of age. Reports show that approximately 4% of women aged 18–22 are bulimic. Females comprise approximately 90% of all anorexia and bulimia cases. Overall, approximately 70 million people worldwide have an eating disorder. Most people who have an eating disorders suffer from the illness for 6 to 10 years.

ANOREXIA

Anorexia is an eating disorder that mainly affects adolescents (most often, girls). People with this disorder have an intense fear of gaining weight and therefore limit the food they eat. Typically, a person with anorexia has an extremely low body weight and a strong refusal to maintain a normal, healthy body weight. The body image of a person with anorexia is usually highly distorted— he or she lives in extreme fear of becoming fat, and is usually unable to recognize that he or she is thin, even dangerously underweight (Figure 7.1).

Anorexia is a way of using food to feel "in control" when dealing with a tough situation. For example, someone may be overwhelmed by his or her parents' divorce, a situation that he or she has no control over. Thus, by starving themselves, people with anorexia feel as though they are exerting control over their lives. There is no single cause of anorexia, and, in fact, the condition may be caused by a number of factors. This disorder often runs in families. Anorexia can be a result of genetics alone. If a person with anorexia has a mother or sister with anorexia, he or she is more likely to develop the disorder. Often, family members criticize a person's body and place a lot of importance on his or her appearance and diet. Another factor contributing to the development of anorexia is the culture of the United States, which places a lot of value on extreme thinness. A person with anorexia has low self-esteem, which results in feeling bad about himself or herself and hating the way he or she looks.

Several signs may indicate that a person has anorexia. These are often behavioral in nature, and include:

1. Loss of a lot of weight;

2. Often focusing on and talking about weight;

3. Moving food around his or her plate, but not eating it;

4. Refusing to eat in front of other people;

5. Using extreme means to lose weight, such as laxatives or diet pill abuse or exercising excessively;

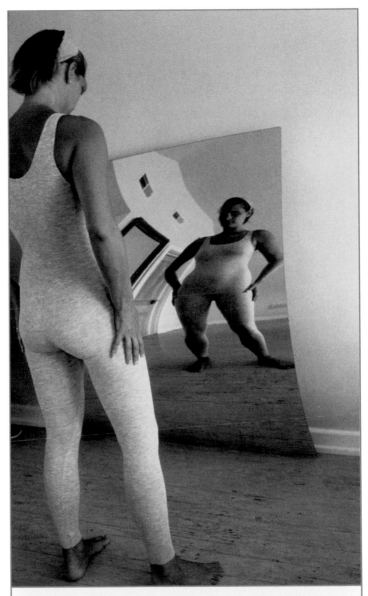

Figure 7.1 Many times, people with eating disorders do not see a "true" image of themselves. When looking into a mirror, these people only see a large, fat stomach and heavy thighs. In reality, they could be so thin that they look like a walking skeleton; only in their heads are they fat.

6. Weighing oneself too often;

7. Acting moody or being depressed.

Anorexia can lead to serious health problems and ultimately affects the entire body (Figure 7.2). The following is a short list of possible complications:

1. Inability to think clearly, moodiness, irritability, fainting;

2. Hair becoming thin and brittle;

3. Low blood pressure, fluttering of the heart, and heart failure;

4. Anemia;

5. Muscle weakness, osteoporosis;

6. Kidney stones, kidney failure;

7. Constipation;

8. In women, lack of menstrual period;

9. Bruising easily, developing dry skin and brittle nails.

BULIMIA

Bulimia is a disease characterized by episodes of binge eating followed by purging (self-induced, deliberate vomiting). This process happens quickly; often the episode of binging and purging happens over 15 to 30 minutes. In addition to purging, bulimic patients misuse laxatives, water pills, and often exercise excessively. This type of behavior may occur approximately 2 to 3 times per week for 3 months. The fear of gaining weight is similar to that experienced by someone who has anorexia. People with bulimia feel an overwhelming need to lose weight, and most are intensely dissatisfied with their bodies. Usually, binging and purging are done in secret, often because bulimics feel ashamed and disgusted with themselves.

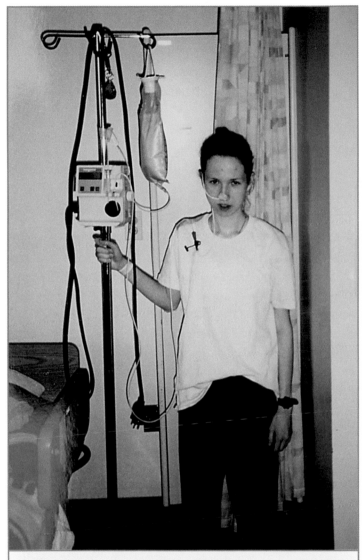

Figure 7.2 The young woman in this picture is anorexic, and has become so malnourished that she must be connected to a heart monitor and receive nutrition through an intravenous line into her body. With medical treatment, her body will likely recover; more important, though, her mind needs to recover so she can see what she is doing to herself and understand what will happen if she continues to starve herself.

The signs and symptoms of bulimia are similar to those of anorexia. Other signs may include binge eating and inappropriate use of diuretics or laxatives. Cavities or gum infections may develop, or the enamel of the teeth may show signs of being stripped off, because of the frequent exposure to stomach acid.

BODY DYSMORPHIC DISORDER (BDD)

BDD is an obsessive-compulsive disorder that leads someone to have a preoccupation with what he or she perceives as a flaw in his or her appearance. Most frequently, the head and

JEN

About 6 months ago, I realized that my daughter Jen had an eating disorder. I began to notice that during dinner she would not really eat; she just pushed her food around on her plate. She exercised all the time, even when she was sick. She became extremely thin; her hair was brittle and thinning. Jen was moody, lashing out one minute and crying the next. I did not know how to help her at all. At first, I really did not do anything because I was frightened to do so—I did not want to put any more stress on her. Then, one day at school, she passed out. The doctors in the emergency room said she needed help, and recommended a program that would keep her in a treatment hospital for 1 month. It killed me inside to do this to her, but after reading and hearing about the possible outcomes of this disorder, such as death, I knew it had to be done and it was the right thing.

Even though Jen was angry with me for a long time, she finally realized that she was slowly killing herself, and eventually she thanked me. She still sees a psychiatrist for her eating disorder, and may have to do so for a long time. She is safe and healthy again, but the road to recovery for this disorder is a rocky one.

BULIMIA

I don't really know how it happened. It had been a very bad weekend and I had come home, screaming at my mother in the car the whole way. I walked inside, slammed the door, headed for the fridge and took out a frozen cheese ravioli dinner, even though I really wasn't hungry. I microwaved it, grew impatient, and ate it half frozen. And then I felt sick. I could feel the slushy tomato sauce rotting in my stomach. And I wanted to throw up.

It was here that it dawned on me that I didn't have to hope to throw up, that I could get rid of the food if I wanted to. I didn't have to suffer for my foolishness. The idea started to take root and I remembered hearing friends tell me how they had made themselves throw up when they were sick before, and I remembered a book where someone had taken the wrong medication and had to get rid of it. And I thought it must be easy. So I went into the bathroom, tucked my hair behind my ears, leaned over the toilet, took a big breath, and stuck two fingers down my throat.

The next morning, I had a bowl of ice cream, and as I sat there feeling stupid for eating ice cream in the morning, I remembered what had happened the night before, so I went and got rid of it. And the next day it was the same thing, and the day after. Until I was doing it every day several times a day. And I thought it was wonderful. I had found a way to erase my mistakes. I could "get rid" of that which I didn't want once I was through with it.

The doctors say this is why I am sitting in this hospital room. This is why I am dehydrated and have been throwing up blood. I will get better, but it will be a slow process. My doctors tell me that I will be in the hospital for a few weeks to get better physically, and then I will have to go to therapy to learn how to talk about my problems.

BODY DYSMORPHIC DISORDER

I hate my body. My nose is too big, my breasts are too small. I am not old enough to consent for surgery myself, but once I turn 18, I will have surgery to correct my ugly nose and to make my breasts bigger. Because of these problems, I cannot get a date with any boys. Once I get these things fixed, I think I am going to have more self-esteem. I mean, how can someone with a big bump on her nose like herself? I do not even want friends right now; I know they will not accept me.

My family tells me all the time that I look great. My nose is perfect, and my weight is good and healthy. I don't believe them. Why should I? They are my family and are supposed to say nice things about me. I know things are not all right. Every time I look in the mirror, all I see are ugly pieces of me. I will change them as soon as I am able to.

face are the primary focus, although any part of the body might be seen as defective. A person with BDD may obsess about acne on the face, too much facial or body hair, too little hair on the head, or having nose, eyes, or feet that are sized or shaped "wrong."

When someone suffers from BDD, his or her social, academic, and professional life may be impaired. When symptoms of BDD are severe, a person might steer clear of social situations altogether, isolating him- or herself from family and friends. The symptoms of this disorder are not easy to notice. Someone who has BDD can easily fool loved ones and friends. Common symptoms include repetitive checking of the perceived flaw in a mirror, avoidance of being photographed, or wearing certain clothes to camouflage an imagined defect. Individuals diagnosed with this disorder may undergo multiple medical procedures (plastic surgery) to correct the perceived flaw.

HEALTH RISKS ASSOCIATED WITH DIET PILL ABUSE

There are health concerns associated with the overuse or abuse of any drug. Abuse can occur with any over-the-counter or prescription drug, including weight loss products. Some of those health concerns are discussed here.

Laxatives and Diuretics

Many people abuse laxatives and diuretics in an effort to control weight. Laxatives work by stimulating nerve endings in the bowel, prompting the release of water from the colon. The idea is that laxatives help food pass more quickly through the body, before calories can be absorbed. The only way that laxatives help you lose weight, however, is by ridding your body of the weight of the water that is lost. This is often referred to as "water weight," and it is weight that comes right back as soon as you start to drink.

Abuse of laxatives can lead to a number of health problems, including imbalances in the levels of minerals (electrolytes) in the body, which can lead to dehydration, tremors, weakness, blurry vision, and kidney damage. Laxatives can also change the way nerve endings in the colon work, which can cause the laxative abuser to need more laxatives to have a bowel movement. Other problems with the digestive system that can result from laxative abuse include an increased risk of colon infection (resulting from a loss of the protective cover that lines the colon), rectal pain, gas, and severe constipation. Finally, laxative abuse may lead to both cancerous and noncancerous tumors in the bowel.

Diuretics cause the body to release excess fluids. They are used to help people with congestive heart failure and high blood pressure, as excess fluid makes heart failure and high blood pressure worse. When someone does not have one of these conditions, the only thing diuretics do is help shed water weight. In general, laxatives and diuretics cause only small amounts of weight to be lost. As weight loss agents, they are not effective.

Abuse of diuretics can lead to problems similar to those resulting from laxative abuse. These include imbalances of certain minerals in the body. Of particular concern is potassium, which is needed at certain concentrations for the heart to pump correctly. Not having enough potassium in the body can lead to an irregular heartbeat, which can result in death. Kidney damage and dehydration are other health risks associated with diuretic abuse.

Amphetamine Abuse

Long-term amphetamine abuse results in many damaging effects, not least of which is addiction. Chronic abusers exhibit symptoms that can include violent behavior, anxiety, confusion, and insomnia. They also can display a number of psychotic features, including paranoia, auditory hallucinations, mood disturbances, and delusions (for example, the sensation of insects creeping on the skin). The paranoia can result in homicidal as well as suicidal thoughts.

USE OF THE BLACK MARKET TO OBTAIN DIET PILLS

Abuse of diet pills is a problem not only due to the concern about the health effects, but also because laws can be broken in the process. Obviously, it is easier to abuse drugs that are more readily available—for example, an over-the-counter laxative—but it can be surprisingly easy to obtain diet pills that require a prescription . . . if one is willing to risk the dangers of dealing with the "black market."

The term *black market*, in this case, applies to a source of prescription drugs other than a retail store or a corner pharmacy (which are regulated by the government). Anyone can easily perform a search on the Internet for "diet pills." The results of this kind of search reveal many Websites that sell drugs without a prescription. Many Websites that say "The Best Diet Pills for Sale," "Buy Phentermine Cheap," or "Cheap Diet Pills," can be located in seconds. If someone wishes to try losing weight using diet pills, they can get the pills easily, and—very often—cheaply.

However, using the Internet to purchase "diet pills" can lead to devastating outcomes. If a person buys and uses diet pills that contain the ingredient phenylpropanolamine (an agent that has been taken off the market), he or she can easily have a stroke. The pills that are sent after purchase online might be sugar pills; they might not even contain the drug that was advertised. If a person is caught buying illegal drugs over the Internet, he or she may face prosecution and possibly even jail. In short, using the Internet or another nonreputable source to acquire diet pills is a high-risk, often no-win, situation.

8

Healthy Ways to Lose Weight and Maintain Weight Loss

The focus of this book to this point has been using drugs, both prescription and over-the-counter, as an aid to losing weight. Before drugs are used, however, other steps must be taken to begin the weight loss process. The first is to assess a patient's weight by calculating his or her BMI and measuring his or her waist circumference (as described in Chapter 1). After determining these values, the next step is to figure out the safest methods for that person to achieve weight loss. Finally, strategies for maintaining weight loss over a long time must be established. Obesity is a lifelong disease and successful treatment involves a lifetime of weight control.

WEIGHT MANAGEMENT

Effective weight control involves many techniques including diet modification, physical activity, and behavior therapy. Generally, doctors and health-care providers recommend that a person looking to lose weight attempt these strategies before considering drug therapy and surgery. Treatment strategies should encourage weight loss and long-term weight control.

There are several ways to begin the weight loss process. Modifying diet and increasing physical activity can influence obesity-related risk factors (when weight affects the heart, for example).

Recommended changes in diet not only modify how many calories someone takes in, but also reduce fat, cholesterol, and sodium found in the person's diet. How much a person exercises is important because it not only helps with weight loss, but also weight maintenance. In addition, exercise can prevent and sometimes even reverse some of the damage done when a person has developed weight-related health problems (for example, high blood pressure). Weight loss should also take into account the needs of the patient. Overall, treatment of overweight and obesity is a commitment that must be taken seriously by both the patient and the health-care professional.

DIETARY THERAPY

People who are overweight or obese should start off by setting a goal for their weight loss. Calorie intake should be reduced by 500 to 1,000 calories per day. This can be done in a number of ways. Simply cutting out one to two sodas a day, for example, may reduce calories; some people switch to diet soda and find that they can shed pounds. This reduction in calories can produce a one- to two-pound weight loss per week. Daily reductions of more than 1,000 calories are not recommended. A person who adopts such extreme calorie reduction will most likely end up in diet failure. He or she may feel so hungry (because of diet restrictions) with the first week or two of dieting, that he or she may simply stop dieting and go back to previous eating habits.

In adjusting a person's diet, it is important to assess the individual's food preferences and make modifications from there. If someone loves to eat chocolate chip cookies, suggesting a low-fat version may be the first step—keeping in mind that reducing fat without reducing calories will not result in weight loss. An overweight or obese person must realize that long-term changes in the diet will lead to long-term weight loss and weight management.

A number of educational efforts can also be undertaken to help an overweight or obese person lose weight. These include:

1. Learning how to read nutrition labels (Figure 8.1). This can help a person determine how many calories a particular food item has and also understand how much fat, carbohydrate, and protein is contained in a food.

2. Learning new strategies for purchasing foods (for example, buying low-calorie foods).

3. Learning methods for food preparation that incorporate lower amounts of oil and fat (for example, using margarine instead of butter or oil to prepare fried chicken, or baking instead of frying).

4. Encouraging a person to drink more water. People— even those who are not trying to lose weight—should be in the habit of drinking 6 to 8 8-ounce glasses of water every day.

5. Learning how to choose correct portion sizes.

6. Learning to substitute low-calorie snacks to help curb the appetite (for example, eating celery and carrot sticks instead of filling up on potato chips).

7. Encouraging a limit on alcohol consumption, because alcohol (beer, wine, and other hard liquors) is high in calories.

There are many national organizations that may be of assistance in helping people lose weight and maintain weight loss; Weight Watchers is one example. In addition, there are a number of "fad diets" for weight loss, which include the Atkins® Diet, South Beach Diet™, and Mediterranean Diet. The main appeal of these diets is that they claim to produce fast weight loss. On the other hand, diets such as the one Weight Watchers recommends helps a person lose weight over approximately 6 months. Studies have found that even though "fad diets" are able to help bring about weight loss

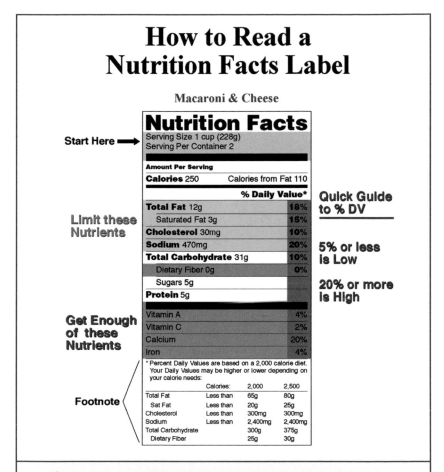

How to Read a
Nutrition Facts Label

Macaroni & Cheese

Start Here ➡

Nutrition Facts
Serving Size 1 cup (228g)
Serving Per Container 2

Amount Per Serving

Calories 250   Calories from Fat 110

Limit these Nutrients

	% Daily Value*
Total Fat 12g	**18%**
Saturated Fat 3g	**15%**
Cholesterol 30mg	**10%**
Sodium 470mg	**20%**
Total Carbohydrate 31g	**10%**
Dietary Fiber 0g	**0%**
Sugars 5g	
Protein 5g	

Get Enough of these Nutrients

Vitamin A	4%
Vitamin C	2%
Calcium	20%
Iron	4%

Quick Guide to % DV

5% or less is Low

20% or more is High

* Percent Daily Values are based on a 2,000 calorie diet.
Your Daily Values may be higher or lower depending on
your calorie needs:

Footnote

		Calories:	2,000	2,500
Total Fat	Less than		65g	80g
Sat Fat	Less than		20g	25g
Cholesterol	Less than		300mg	300mg
Sodium	Less than		2,400mg	2,400mg
Total Carbohydrate			300g	375g
Dietary Fiber			25g	30g

Figure 8.1 A nutrition label can look daunting if you have not read one before. Consumers should pay attention to certain aspects of the label when determining the health content of the food. First, it is important to notice the number of servings in a package. For example, you might be used to eating the whole package of macaroni and cheese, but you can tell from the label that there are 2 servings per package. This information is important when reading the rest of the label. Next, look at the number of calories per serving. Even more important is the total fat and saturated fat content in the food. Saturated fat is the "bad" fat and having more of this makes the food even more unhealthy. If you eat all of the macaroni and cheese, you have doubled the serving size and thus doubled the calories and fat.

quickly, the amount of weight lost after six months for both kinds of diets was the same. Overall, it is very hard to stick to "fad diets" that restrict one type of food (for example, carbohydrates). Weight Watchers allows a person to eat foods (in moderation) that can cause weight gain, and even offers recipes that are low fat but taste good.

PHYSICAL ACTIVITY

Increasing physical activity produces direct and indirect benefits. Simply exercising for 30 minutes, three to five times per week, will assist with weight loss. Increased exercise leads to increased energy expenditure and plays a large role in weight loss. Continued exercise most importantly leads to weight maintenance. Moreover, exercise reduces the risk of heart disease more than does weight loss alone. Increased physical activity helps decrease the risk of heart disease and type II diabetes, which go hand-in-hand with being overweight or obese. Also, exercise can prevent a decrease in muscle mass, something that is often seen in overweight or obese people.

Many people have difficult finding the motivation to exercise. Simply starting an exercise routine requires a lot of support from loved ones or a support group to offer encouragement. It is also important to realize that before you start an exercise regimen you may need to contact your doctor for medical clearance. Extremely overweight people need to start low and go slow, beginning with simple exercises and gradually increasing the complexity and intensity of their exercise. This approach is the best strategy for achieving successful weight loss and weight maintenance.

Some physical activities can be very simple to add to the daily routine—taking the stairs instead of the elevator, or walking instead of driving, are good examples. Eventually, a person can add more strenuous activities to his or her routine, such as speed walking, bicycling, tennis, and jumping rope.

Table 8.1 Examples of Moderate Physical Activity

HOUSEHOLD CHORES	SPORTS AND ATHLETICS
Washing and waxing a car for 45–60 minutes	Playing volleyball for 45–60 minutes
Pushing a stroller 1 1/2 miles in 30 minutes	Playing touch football for 45 minutes
Walking 2 miles in 30 minutes	Shooting hoops for 30 minutes
Shoveling snow for 15 minutes	Dancing for 30 minutes
Gardening for 30–45 minutes	Jumping rope for 15 minutes

Adapted from the National Heart, Lung, and Blood Institute Guidelines. Available online at *http://www.nhlbi.gov/health/pulic/heart/obesity/lose_wt/phy_act.htm.*

Team sports, such as volleyball or softball, are other options for increasing activity levels. A person engaging in any strenuous exercise should take caution at first, so as to not strain the body and cause injury. Table 8.1 lists some activities that can help a person expend energy and burn off calories.

Reducing sedentary time—that is, time spent watching TV, playing video games, or using the computer—is another way to achieve weight loss. Getting up and walking is very easy to do! A person who takes public transportation can get off one stop early and walk the extra distance. He or she can park farther away from the shopping mall entrance and walk across the parking lot, then walk up the stairs instead of using an elevator or escalator. Of course, it is important to find safe places to perform these activities. When a safe place cannot be identified, exercising at home is one option for increasing physical activity. Using a treadmill or stationary bicycle will allow a person to exercise at home. Also, there are a number of exercise videos that incorporate walking in place as a home workout. Some of these are the equivalent of a 3-mile walk! People should be encouraged to plan their exercise one week in advance. This allows them to budget the time necessary to exercise. In addition, people should keep a diary of physical activity.

Overall, a person should aim to burn about 150 calories per workout to start; this leads to an expenditure of 450 calories per week. The goal number of calories to burn is 1,000 per week. This would equal walking 30 minutes a day or one hour 3 times per week. Specific recommendations have been made by the National Institutes of Health with regard to exercise:

1. For a beginner, exercise should start off very light: standing more (ironing and cooking will fulfill this).

2. Light activity is achieved though slow walking, house cleaning, or babysitting.

3. Moderate exercise is defined as walking a mile in 15 minutes, bicycling, or dancing.

4. High exercise is achieved by jogging for 10 minutes or playing basketball or soccer.

Other activities should be introduced slowly. Warming up muscles before exercise (slow walking before speed walking, for example) and stretching after exercise is important. Exercises that increase flexibility should be encouraged. Both muscle-building (for example, weight lifting) and aerobic (for example, walking or jogging) exercise should be performed.

BEHAVIOR THERAPY

Ultimately, changes in behavior lead to successful weight loss more than anything else. Changes in behavior may have a much larger impact on weight loss than once thought. High stress can lead to overeating. People who are in a period of emotional turmoil (such as the loss of a loved one) often eat to cope with their problems. Beyond dieting and physical activity, stress-reducing techniques and learning how to cope with emotional problems (with the help of a support group or counselor) are additional steps to losing weight. All of these changes can lead improved weight management. A doctor or other health-care professional can suggest other ways that a person can achieve weight loss. Assessing a person's motivation for losing weight must be included in this process. Encouragement is a key component to weight loss.

Being obese or overweight is not new for most of these patients. Obese people are often victims of shame and hurtful comments from others. A health-care professional should understand the patient's weight problem (when and how he or she puts on weight). Among the main concerns are the health risks that go along with being overweight or obese. Weight loss and maintenance of weight is not an easy task. A health-care professional can realize this and help the patient achieving his or her weight loss goals. The person looking to lose weight must realize, however, that losing weight is a commitment that he or she must work at to be successful.

Sometimes a person on a weight loss program finds that he or she is not losing weight. There are several questions a person in this situation can ask to understand what may be happening. Has the person been under stress? Did he or she sustain an injury that interferes with or prevents exercise? Has the person become bored with his or her routine? Answering questions like these can help a person make adjustments that will help him or her achieve his or her goals. Sometimes, a person limiting his or her caloric intake feels deprived and eats more, especially fat-filled foods. Making dietary changes that are small and easier to adopt (for example, eating with a smaller plate than usual) may be the solution.

When weight loss programs incorporate low-fat diets, reduced caloric intake, increased physical activity, and behavior therapy, an individual is more likely to maintain his or her weight loss. For all people looking to lose weight, this is the first step that must be taken. When they are necessary, weight loss drugs and surgery are the next logical steps. Drugs and surgery cannot be used by all people who want to lose weight, however. Willpower, learning how to lose weight safely, and understanding that the weight loss process has its ups and downs are all needed for successful weight loss and management.

WEIGHT LOSS SURGERY

When a patient is faced with severe obesity and has multiple health problems because of it, weight loss surgery might be necessary. Doctors will consider whether the person would live for another five years if he or she does not lose a great deal of weight quickly, as through surgery. There are many risks associated with weight-loss surgery; the risks may outweigh the benefits.

The National Heart, Lung and Blood Institute (NHLBI) has established criteria for people considering weight loss surgery. However, many people who do not fit the NHLBI criteria have weight loss surgery anyway. Often these patients cannot deal with the societal issues that go with being overweight; others undergo the surgery for health and cosmetic reasons.

For people who are severely obese (defined as a BMI of 40 or greater or 35 or greater with other health problems), surgery (often called "stomach stapling") may be the only option. Surgery should not be offered until diet modification and weight loss drugs have failed. This type of surgery has not been performed for many years and there are unknown risks to this invasive procedure. There is a high risk of complications during the surgery itself, and after, which can result in

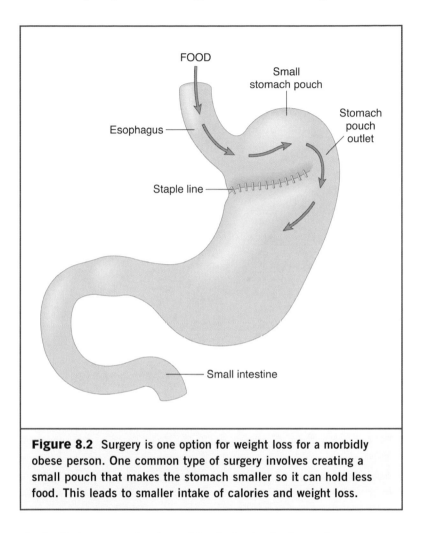

FOOD

Small
stomach pouch

Stomach
pouch
outlet

Esophagus

Staple line

Small intestine

Figure 8.2 Surgery is one option for weight loss for a morbidly obese person. One common type of surgery involves creating a small pouch that makes the stomach smaller so it can hold less food. This leads to smaller intake of calories and weight loss.

death. Patients can develop a blood clot in the leg or lung, or develop an infection.

Recovery time from this operation can last anywhere from six to eight weeks. As soon as the patient can begin to eat solid food, he or she must learn how to eat again. The stomach has essentially become a small pouch and cannot hold the same amount of food that it used to (Figure 8.2). Patients must eat a healthier diet after this surgery; they are much less able to tolerate a diet high in fat. Overall, weight-loss surgery should be considered a last option after all other alternatives have failed.

A program to lose weight has to consider a patient's readiness to lose weight. Weight loss is not an easy process. A person has to have reasons and motivation for weight loss. He or she must have the support of family and friends. The risks and benefits of weight loss must be explained and understood. If all of these items are part of a weight loss program, a successful journey can begin.

Diet Pills: The Future

The quest for the perfect weight loss drug continues as the prevalence of obesity in the United States and other industrialized
countries rises. Why has it been so difficult for drug manufacturers
to develop the "perfect" diet pill? One reason is that the causes of
obesity are not fully understood, so it is difficult for researchers to
select a specific target in the body to focus on when studying
potential drugs. Safety is another challenge; most drugs that cause
weight loss have negative effects on metabolism and other body
processes. Another important reason many diet drugs have failed is
that they have been intended for short-term treatment only. Most
people gain the weight back as soon as they stop taking the drug.
A weight loss agent that provides long-term weight maintenance
would have a better chance of being successful. In summary, the
perfect diet pill would cause rapid weight loss and long-term weight
maintenance with little or no serious side effects.

RIMONABANT

Rimonabant (brand name: Acomplia®) is currently under development. This drug has shown early evidence that it may be able to
counteract obesity and help people quit smoking. Rimonabant is
part of a new class of drugs called endocannabinoids, which work by
blocking the same pathways in the brain that give people who smoke
marijuana the "munchies." Scientists have found a way to block the
cannabinoid receptors in the brain in the hopes of stopping food
cravings. In trials of the drug, patients were treated with rimonabant or placebo (sugar pill) for one year. Almost half of the patients

receiving rimonabant lost 10% of their body weight by the end of the trial (for example, a 220-lb [100-kg] person lost at least 22 lbs [10 kg]). People receiving rimonabant lost significantly more weight than people in the placebo group. People on rimonabant also appeared to have improved cholesterol levels, and people with diabetes appeared to have better blood sugar control, although this requires further study.

Specific adverse effects of rimonabant have not yet been released to the public, although the company that makes the drug reports that their incidence is low. Pending the completion of more safety and efficacy studies, rimonabant is expected to be available in the United States in the next couple of years. This drug may prove to be especially ideal for obese individuals who smoke, since it should help with both problems.

AXOKINE®

Axokine® is another new drug under development. Axokine is a synthetic (man-made) chemical that mimics a hormone produced in the brain that is responsible for protecting the body from injury. Axokine was initially developed as a treatment for Lou Gehrig's disease, but researchers noticed that

DRUG TESTING

Diet drugs that are in development take years to be approved and marketed in the United States. First, these compounds are studied in the laboratory. Then, they are tested in animals. The next step is to be tested in people. There are three rounds of study—called Phases I, II, and III trials—to establish safety and effectiveness of the drug in humans. Drugs that are in Phase III trials are closest to approval and are usually available in the United States within a couple of years if they prove to be safe and effective. Drugs in Phase II trials are a little further behind in the approval process.

patients who were taking this drug lost weight. Researchers then turned their attention to studying this drug for weight loss.

Axokine affects the leptin pathway in the brain. As discussed in Chapter 2, leptin is a chemical messenger that tells the brain when the body has had enough to eat. People who are obese may not respond appropriately to this messenger, thus they may not realize they are full. Axokine apparently helps these individuals respond appropriately to leptin.

The main side effects associated with Axokine are nausea and cough. Unlike the other drugs discussed in this book, Axokine is an injection, not a pill. Axokine must be given with a needle, which may cause some pain at the site where it is injected. Axokine is currently being studied in a Phase III trial for weight loss. If Axokine proves to be safe and effective, it should be available in the United States within a few years.

P57

Scientists found that the *Hoodia* cactus contained a previously unknown molecule, P57, that may produce weight loss. P57 is

JACKIE

Jackie is a 46-year-old woman who weighed 180 pounds and was only five feet, four inches tall. She read about rimonabant, a drug that was being investigated in clinical trials for weight loss. Jackie was able to participate in a clinical trial and took this drug for one year. She lost 30 pounds during that time.

As soon as the trial ended and she could no longer get the drug, she regained the 30 pounds that she lost. She is waiting for the drug to be approved by the FDA so she can begin to take it again.

(Adapted from *Newsweek*, August 23, 2004, p. 46.)

the active ingredient that scientists have isolated from the *Hoodia gordonii* cactus. As mentioned in Chapter 6, *Hoodia* is a cactus that grows in extremely hot climates, specifically in the African Kalahari Desert (Figure 9.1). The stems and roots of the *Hoodia* cactus were supposedly consumed by the San Kalahari bushmen for thousands of years to stave off hunger during long hunting trips. *Hoodia* gives a sense of satiety (fullness). The San Bushmen report no side effects from the use of the cactus; however, this requires further study.

A large drug manufacturer has decided to study this molecule and formulate it into a drug if it proves to be safe and effective. As an aside, the San Bushmen of the Kalahari desert are currently impoverished and oppressed. If P57 becomes a money-making drug in developed countries, it may mean a better life for people of this tribe, since they will receive royalties (money) when the drug is sold. This drug is very early in the research process and it will be several years before it could be available in the United States.

CHOLESCYSTOKIN BOOSTERS AND NEUROPEPTIDE Y INHIBITORS

As discussed in Chapter 3, there are many hormones present in different concentrations in the body. Either increasing or decreasing these hormones can assist with weight loss. Two hormones in particular, cholecystokinin (CCK) and cholecyctokinin boosters, are currently under investigation as possible weight loss agents. CCK is a naturally occurring appetite suppressant.

A neuropeptide Y (NYP) inhibitor is also being investigated as a possible weight loss drug. NYP inhibitors block a potent chemical, neuropeptide Y, which is an appetite stimulant.

THE FUTURE OF WEIGHT LOSS DRUGS

These days, there is a lot of pressure to "look good." As a result, many young people who are overweight think they should not laugh, smile, or do anything that might draw attention to

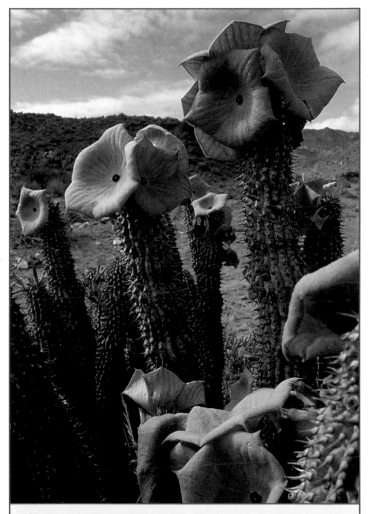

Figure 9.1 The *Hoodia gordonii* plant is a flowering cactus that is native to the African Kalahari Desert. The San Kalahari Bushmen supposedly consumed the stems and roots of this plant for centuries to stave off hunger while on long hunting trips. Scientists believe they have isolated the active ingredient (ingredient that exerts the effects of appetite suppression) from the *Hoodia* plant. Scientists have named the active ingredient P57 and are currently working on making this ingredient into a drug that can be used for weight loss.

them. Often, overweight and obese individuals are depressed and feel there is no hope that they can ever lose weight. These people resort to diet pills as their only way to lose excess weight. They feel that if they take more diet pills, they do not have to "watch what they eat" or exercise. The health and legal ramifications of diet pill abuse are never considered. What these individuals do not realize is that weight loss and mainte- nance need to become a way of life. Abuse of diet pills is not the way to lose weight; the resulting weight loss is temporary and abuse of these agents can lead to death.

The quest for the perfect diet pill is far from over. Readers should use reputable Internet sites and other sources to keep abreast of new developments. In most cases, diet pills will only be recommended for obese individuals who fall into certain risk-based categories. All drugs have side effects; the benefits must always outweigh the risks when you decide to take these pills.

1 National Heart, Lung and Blood Institute (NHLBI). "Clinical Guidelines on the Identification, Evaluation, and Treatment of Overweight and Obesity in Adults." Available online at *http://www.nhlbi.nih.gov/guidelines/obesity/ob_home.htm.*

2 Ibid.

3 American Obesity Association. Available online at *http://www.obesity.org.*

4 Ibid.

5 Weintraub, M., et al. "Long term Weight Control Study Conclusions," *Clinical Pharmacology Therapeutics* 51(1992): 619–633.

6 Kernan, W. N., et al. "Phenypropanolamine and the Risk of Hemorrhagic Stroke." *New England Journal of Medicine* 343(2000): 1826–1832.

7 American Obesity Association. "AOA Fact Sheets, Consumer Protection: Weight Management Products & Services." Available online at *http://www.obesity.org/subs/fastfacts/Obesity_Consumer_Protect.shtml.*

Bibliography

Books and Articles

Baskin, M. L., H. K. Ahluwalia, and K. Resnicow. "Obesity Intervention Among African-American Children and Adolescents." *Pediatric Clinics of North America* 48(4) (2001): 1027–1039.

Blumenthal, M., et al. *The Complete German Commission E Herbal Monographs: Therapeutic Guide to Herbal Medicines.* Austin: American Botanical Council, 1998.

Bray, G. A. "A Concise Review on the Therapeutics of Obesity." *Nutrition* 16(10)(2000): 953–960.

———. "Obesity." *Harrison's principles of internal medicine,* 14th ed., eds. K. J. Isselbacher, J. D. Wilson, J. B. Martin, D. L. Kasper, S. L. Hauser, and D. L. Longo. New York: McGraw-Hill, 1998, pp. 454–462.

DeEugenio, D., and M. L. Smith. "Management of Thyroid Disorders." *Pharmacy Times.* June 2004.

Forman, S. F. "Eating Disorders: Epidemiology, pathogenesis, and clinical features." *Uptodate,* ed. S. F. Forman. Wellesley, MA: Uptodate, 2004.

Glazer, Gary. "Long-term Pharmacotherapy of Obesity 2000: A Review of Efficacy and Safety." *Archives of Internal Medicine* 161(2001): 1814–1824.

Jellin, Jeff M. *Natural Medicine Comprehensive Database 2004,* 6th ed. Stockton: Therapeutic Research Center, 2004.

Krotkiewski, M. "Thyroid Hormones and Treatment of Obesity." *International Journal of Obesity and Related Metabolic Disorders* 24(suppl 2)(2000): S116–119.

Labib, M. "The Investigation and Management of Obesity." *Journal of Clinical Pathology* 56(2003): 17–25.

Martikainen, P. T., and M. G. Marmot. "Socioeconomic differences in weight gain and determinants and consequences of coronary risk factors." American Journal of Clinical Nutrition 69(4)(1999): 719–726.

McEvoy, Gerald K. *AHFS Drug Information 2002.* Bethesda: American Society of Health-Systems Pharmacists, 2002.

Mundy, Alicia. "Weight-loss Wars: A Spate of Deaths and a Raft of Lawsuits Over Diet Drugs." *U.S. News & World Report.* February 15, 1999, pp. 42–44.

Gennaro, Alfanso, ed. "Adrenergic and Adrenergic Blocking Drugs." *Remington: The Science and Practice of Pharmacy.* Baltimore: Lippincott Williams & Wilkins, 2003, pp. 1322–1328.

Sothern, M. S., and S. T. Gordon. "Prevention of Obesity in Young Children: A Critical Challenge for Medical Professionals." *Clinical Pediatrics* 42(2003): 101–111.

St. Peter, John V., and Mehmood A. Khan. "Obesity." *Pharmacotherapy: A Pathophysiologic Approach*, 5th ed. New York: McGraw-Hill, 2002, pp. 2543–2563.

Underwood, A., and J. Adler. "What You Don't Know About Fat." *Newsweek.* August 23, 2004, p. 40.

Websites

http://www.obesity.org
American Obesity Association

http://www.anred.com
Anorexia Nervosa and Related Eating Disorders, Inc. (ANRED)

http://www.healthyweightforum.org
Healthy Weight Forum

http://www.theheart.org/
The Heart.org

www.mcdonalds.com
McDonald's

http://www.pharma-lexicon.com
Medi-Lexicon

http://www.nhlbi.nih.gov/guidelines/obesity/ob_home.htm
National Heart, Lung, and Blood Institute (NHLBI). "Clinical Guidelines on the Identification, Evaluation, and Treatment of Overweight and Obesity in Adults"

http://www.nhlbi.nih.gov/about/oei/
Obesity Education Initiative

http://www.nimh.nih.gov/publicat/eatingdisorders.cfm
National Institute of Mental Health (NIMH). "Eating Disorders: Facts About Eating Disorders and the Search for Solutions"

http://www.4women.gov/
National Women's Health Information Center (NWHIC)

http://ods.od.nih.gov/factsheets/DietarySupplements.asp
Office of Dietary Supplements (National Institutes of Health). "Dietary Supplements: Background Information"

http://www.consumer.gov/weightloss/guidelines.htm
Partnership for Healthy Weight Management. "Voluntary Guidelines for Providers of Weight Loss Products or Services"

http://www.phrma.org
Pharmaceutical Research and Manufacturers of America (PhRMA)

http://www.berkeleywellness.com/
University of California, Berkeley. "Wellness Letter.com; The Newsletter of Nutrition, Fitness, and Self-Care"

http://www.fda.gov/
U.S. Food and Drug Administration (FDA)

http://www.cfsan.fda.gov/~dms/supplmnt.html
U.S. Food and Drug Administration, Center for Food Safety and Applied Nutrition: Dietary Supplements

http://www.cdc.gov
U.S. Centers for Disease Control and Prevention

Further Reading

Agatston, A. *The South Beach Diet.* New York: Random House, 2003.

Beale L., and S. G. Couvillon. *The Complete Idiot's Guide to Weight Loss.* Indianapolis: Alpha Books, 2003.

Beers, M. H., ed. *The Merck Manual of Medical Information,* 2nd Home Edition. New York, NY: Pocketbooks, 2003.

Bralow, L., ed. *The Physician's Desk Reference (PDR) Pocket Guide to Prescription Drugs.* New York: Pocketbooks, 2003.

Griffith, H. W. *The Complete Guide to Prescription and Non-prescription Drugs, 2004 Ed.* New York: Berkley Publishing Group, 2003.

Index

Index

114

Index

Index

About the Authors

Deborah DeEugenio, Pharm.D., B.C.P.S., is a 2001 graduate of the Philadelphia College of Pharmacy at the University of the Sciences (Philadelphia). She completed a residency in Pharmacy Practice at Thomas Jefferson University Hospital (Philadelphia). Dr. DeEugenio is a member of the Temple University School of Pharmacy faculty as a Clinical Assistant Professor and a Certified Antithrombotic Provider and a Board Certified Pharmacotherapy Specialist. Her clinical activity takes place at Jefferson Heart Institute as part of the Jefferson Antithrombotics Therapy Service. The ambulatory clinic serves 400 patients on chronic anticoagulation therapy and provides continuous monitoring and education to these patients. The clinic also provides drug information and pharmacy support to the physicians and other health-care providers at the Institute.

Debra Henn, Pharm.D., is a 2001 graduate of the Philadelphia College of Pharmacy at the University of the Sciences (Philadelphia). She completed a residency in Drug Information at Thomas Jefferson University Hospital (Philadelphia), in conjunction with Bristol-Myers Squibb Company. She now holds a position with Crozer-Chester Medical Center (Upland, PA) as the Clinical Specialist in Drug Information. Dr. Henn is also a part-time adjunct faculty member at Philadelphia College of Pharmacy. Her practice involves the provision of drug information to the medical staff at Crozer, handling various activities related to the Pharmacy and Therapeutics Committee, editing a bimonthly pharmacy newsletter and as a committee member of the Institutional Review Board.

About the Editor

David J. Triggle is a University Professor and a Distinguished Professor in the School of Pharmacy and Pharmaceutical Sciences at the State University of New York at Buffalo. He studied in the United Kingdom and earned his B.Sc. degree in Chemistry from the University of Southampton and a Ph.D. degree in Chemistry at the University of Hull. Following post-doctoral work at the University of Ottawa in Canada and the University of London in the United Kingdom, he assumed a position at the School of Pharmacy at Buffalo. He served as Chairman of the Department of Biochemical Pharmacology from 1971 to 1985 and as Dean of the School of Pharmacy from 1985 to 1995. From 1995 to 2001 he served as the Dean of the Graduate School, and as the University Provost from 2000 to 2001. He is the author of several books dealing with the chemical pharmacology of the autonomic nervous system and drug-receptor interactions, some 400 scientific publications, and has delivered over 1,000 lectures worldwide on his research.

Picture Credits